CORPVS MEDICORVM GRAECORVM SVPPLEMENTVM ORIENTALE

EDIDERVNT

ACADEMIAE BEROLINENSIS HAVNIENSIS LIPSIENSIS

II

GALENI

DE PARTIBVS ARTIS MEDICATIVAE
DE CAVSIS CONTENTIVIS
DE DIAETA IN MORBIS ACVTIS SECVNDVM HIPPOCRATEM
LIBELLORVM VERSIONES ARABICAS

EDIDIT ET IN LINGVAM ANGLICAM VERTIT

MALCOLM LYONS

DE PARTIBVS ARTIS MEDICATIVAE
DE CAVSIS CONTENTIVIS
LIBELLORVM EDITIONES ALTERIVS AB HERMANNO SCHOENE
ALTERIVS A CAROLO KALBFLEISCH CVRATAS

RETRACTAVERVNT

J. KOLLESCH D. NICKEL G. STROHMAIER

BEROLINI IN AEDIBVS ACADEMIAE SCIENTIARVM MCMLXIX

GALEN

ON THE PARTS OF MEDICINE
ON COHESIVE CAUSES
ON REGIMEN IN ACUTE DISEASES IN ACCORDANCE WITH THE THEORIES OF HIPPOCRATES

FIRST EDITION OF THE ARABIC VERSIONS
WITH ENGLISH TRANSLATION
BY

MALCOLM LYONS

THE LATIN VERSIONS OF
ON THE PARTS OF MEDICINE ED. BY H. SCHOENE
AND
ON COHESIVE CAUSES ED. BY K. KALBFLEISCH
REEDITED BY
J. KOLLESCH D. NICKEL G. STROHMAIER

AKADEMIE-VERLAG · BERLIN 1969

Erschienen im Akademie-Verlag GmbH, 108 Berlin, Leipziger Straße 3–4

Lizenznummer: 202 · 100/142/69
Herstellung: IV/2/14 VEB Werkdruck Gräfenhainichen · 2850
Bestellnummer: 2028/14 · ES 7 L, 7 M
90,–

CONTENTS

ABBREVIATIONS

CMG I 1	Hippocratis Indices Librorum, Iusiurandum, Lex etc. ed I. L. Heiberg, Leipzig, Berlin 1927 (Corpus Medicorum Graecorum I 1)
CMG V 9, 1	Galeni In Hippocratis De natura hominis, In Hippocratis De victu acutorum, De diaeta Hippocratis in morbis acutis, edd. J. Mewaldt, G. Helmreich, J. Westenberger, Leipzig, Berlin 1914 (Corpus Medicorum Graecorum V 9, 1)
Helmr.	Galeni De elementis ex Hippocratis sententia libri duo, ed. G. Helmreich, Erlangen 1878
K.	Claudii Galeni Opera omnia, 20 voll., ed. C. G. Kühn, Leipzig 1821–1833, repr. Hildesheim 1964–1965
Kw.	Hippocratis Opera quae feruntur omnia, 2 voll., ed. H. Kühlewein, Leipzig 1894, 1902
L.	Œuvres complètes d'Hippocrate, 10 voll., ed. É. Littré, Paris 1839–1861
Scr. min.	Claudii Galeni Pergameni Scripta minora, 3 voll., edd. J. Marquardt, I. Müller, G. Helmreich, Leipzig 1884, 1891, 1893

PREFACES

De Partibus Artis Medicativae

The Arabic translation of Galen's work, De partibus artis medicativae, appears to have attracted no great amount of attention amongst the bibliographers, of whom Ibn an-Nadīm, Ibn al-Qifṭī and Ḥajjī Khalīfa have all failed to record it. Ibn abī Uṣaibiʿa[1] notes it as: "A tract on the parts of medicine in which medicine is divided up in accordance with various methods of partition and division". The source of this statement is doubtless the *Risāla* of Ḥunain ibn Isḥāq, who, in his list of Galen's productions, writes of the work[2]: "This tract, also, consists of a single section and in it the art of medicine is divided up in various ways. I translated it into Syriac for a man called ʿAlī, known as al-Fayyūm." This note is continued by a gloss which runs: "Ḥunain translated more than half of this work about two months before his death and Isḥāq finished it. The translation was made into Arabic." It might be argued that this final remark merely applies to an Arabic addition by Isḥāq to Ḥunain's Syriac, but this seems sufficiently unlikely to allow it to be discounted here[3]. If it is then assumed that the gloss is referring to a full Arabic translation made both by Ḥunain and by his son Isḥāq, it remains to question whether this is the version presented here.

Before this problem can conclusively be settled, the techniques of stylometry, so ably pioneered in this field by Bergsträßer, must be applied to a far wider range of translation texts than is yet available for study and analysis. At best, in short tracts, the scope for the appli-

---

[1] *Kitāb ʿuyūn al-anbāʾ*, ed. Müller (Cairo 1882), vol. 1, p. 97.

[2] Ed. Bergsträßer, Abhandlungen für die Kunde des Morgenlandes 17, 2, no. 61.

[3] Bergsträßer's recension B quotes this note in an altered form which states definitely that Ḥunain's translation was made into Arabic: – Neue Materialien zu Ḥunain ibn Isḥāq's Galen-Bibliographie, Abhandlungen für die Kunde des Morgenlandes 19, 2, p. 34sq.

cation of such techniques must be limited and the possibility of freakish results can never be discounted, more particularly where translations may have been revised and corrected by a number of scholars. As a result, it has not been thought worth recording a full stylistic analysis of the present text in that, by itself, this could not provide a reliable guide to authorship. However, it may be noted that, on general grounds, it seems unlikely that the present version can be accepted uncritically as a joint work by Ḥunain and Isḥāq. That Ḥunain concerned himself with the text is clear enough both from his own words and from the quantity of explanatory notes in the text introduced by the words: "Ḥunain said"[1]. But the version presented in this edition, though it maintains a reasonable standard of scholarship, appears stylistically inferior to the works of the best Arab translators, amongst whom the place of Ḥunain and Isḥāq is unquestioned. The reader will find instances of oddity of expression, clumsiness of construction, ambiguity and repetitiveness of language that tend to mar the flow of the work[2]. Neither individually nor cumulatively can these be taken as final proof, positive or negative, of authorship, but they must at least be noted as casting doubt on the accuracy of the gloss or on the identification of the version to which it refers with that of the present edition.

The text of this edition is based on a single manuscript, in the Aya Sofya collection in Istanbul (Aya Sofya 3725, 183^b–192^a), which has been noted and described by Ritter and Walzer in their article: "Arabische Übersetzungen griechischer Ärzte in Stambuler Bibliotheken."[3] The tract is dated to the year 456 A. H.–1063 A. D. The copyist, who has not signed his name, writes in a clear but rather coarse hand. He uses few orthographical signs, though *shadda* is sometimes inserted and sentence endings are marked by a stop φ. Diacritical points are added in the majority of cases. There is evidence that the copyist took some care to establish his text, as on one occasion he adds a varia lectio in the margin[4]. He has also been at some pains to insert explanatory notes, attributed to Ḥunain, for which he normally leaves room in his margins.

---

1 pp. 26, 30, 32, 34.

2 As examples may be noted such expressions as: اقل قليل p. 28, l. 26; 32, l. 15. اجزاءها التى هى بحسب المادة التى هى اولى بها p. 44, l. 12.

3 Sitzungsber. d. Preuß. Akad. d. Wissensch., phil.-hist. Klasse, 1934, p. 816, no. 27.

4 p. 30.

De Causis Contentivis

The Arabic translation of Galen's work, De causis contentivis, presents its own immediate problem of nomenclature. The translation was identified by Bergsträßer as the work listed in the *Risāla* of Ḥunain ibn Isḥāq under the title of The Book of The Causes Connected with Disease (*Kitāb al-asbāb al-muttaṣila bi'l-maraḍ*[1]). There seems to be no adequate reason for doubting Bergsträßer's identification, more particularly since the only text with which it could simply be confused, that of Galen's De causis morborum, is proved by a description of its content and context to be the work that Ḥunain lists as the *Kitāb asbāb al-amrāḍ*. Of the *Kitāb al-asbāb al-muttaṣila bi'l-maraḍ* Ḥunain writes: "It consists of a single tract in which he (Galen) mentions the causes connected with disease and that serve to produce it. The account of it is like that of the preceding text."[2] This latter reference is to the work *Kitāb al-asbāb al-bādi'a*, of which Ḥunain writes: "It was translated by Ayyūb (ibn al-Abrash). I have had a Greek manuscript of it with me but I have not had leisure to translate it."

The title given by the present text, *Kitāb al-asbāb al-māsika*, is not to be found in Ḥunain's account, though it is mentioned by Ibn abī Uṣaibiʿa, who lists it amongst works not named in the *Risāla*, though found in translations made "either by Ḥunain or by others"[3]. In the absence of any further evidence, if Bergsträßer's identification is accepted as being correct, it must be assumed that in a version made of the work post-dating the *Risāla* the title was changed to its present form. On the evidence of the heading of the version presented here this translation was made by Ḥunain himself, though this may imply no more than that he revised an existing version made by Ayyūb ibn al-Abrash or, perhaps more likely, that he turned a Syriac version made by Ayyūb into Arabic. Stylistic evidence is of some negative value here, in that the Arabic may be thought of suf-

---

[1] Abhandlungen für die Kunde des Morgenlandes, 17, 2, no. 59.
[2] *Risāla*, ed. Bergsträßer, loc. cit.
[3] *Kitāb ʿuyūn al-anbā'*, ed. Müller (Cairo 1882), vol. 1, p. 103.

ficiently high quality to have been written by Ḥunain, though it is unlikely that this can be proved positively.

The text of the present edition is based on a single Istanbul manuscript, Aya Sofya 3725, 85ᵃ–94ᵃ, of which Ritter and Walzer, who described it in their article "Arabische Übersetzungen griechischer Ärzte in Stambuler Bibliotheken", noted that it is a medical codex containing 218 folios (20×14½ cm)[1]. The text of this particular work is shown by its colophon to have been copied by a certain Khalaf[2] ibn abī Rabīʿ al-Andalusī, "for his own purposes". A note adds virtuously that the text was compared with that of the original, to establish that it was as sound as possible and there are a number of alterations and corrections added to it in the copyist's own hand that go to show that there is some substance in this claim. The text itself is without a date, but a close approximation to it can be given by two other dates in the same codex that are noted by Ritter and Walzer as 456 A. H.–1063 A. D. and 457 A. H.–1064 A. D.

The copyist employs a small but clear script. He normally adds diacritical points, but he uses few orthographical signs, apart from the occasional insertion of the *fatḥatain* ending. He produces the sign φ as an occasional punctuation stop. His text contains a number of grammatical mistakes for which it may be argued that he is responsible. Where these have been emended in this edition this has been noted in the textual Apparatus. It must be stressed, though, that such emendations have been made chiefly for the convenience of readers and it should not be taken as an attempt to prejudice the question of whether or not the translators themselves followed the normal canons of grammatical Arabic.

---

1 Sitzungsber. d. Preuß. Akad. d. Wissensch., phil.-hist. Klasse, 1934, p. 817, no. 28.
2 Ritter & Walzer, p. 841, Ḥalfu.

De Diaeta in Morbis Acutis secundum Hippocratem

In his work De libris propriis Galen twice[1] refers to an account that he wrote of Hippocrates' De diaeta in morbis acutis, which is distinguished from the five sections of his own commentary on this work. A similar text is noted by the Arab bibliographers, Ibn an-Nadīm[2], Ibn abī Uṣaibiʿa[3] and Ibn al-Qifṭī[4], as consisting of a single section. Ḥunain ibn Isḥāq writes of it in his *Risāla*[5]: "This work consists of a single section and Galen's intention in it can be understood from its title. Recently I translated it into Syriac for Bukhtīshūʿ and afterwards I made an Arabic version of it for Muḥammad ibn Mūsā." Such a work was published in Latin by Caius and in Greek by Chartier, though it was found only in a truncated version and was attributed to Galen on the authority of the copyists of its two extant manuscripts. Westenberger, who edited the Greek text in the series Corpus Medicorum Graecorum[6], traces its history fully and quotes the arguments that have been advanced against its authenticity, prompted both by its style and its subject matter. Westenberger's conclusion is that, though such doubts have always existed, the fact that his text passes in its manuscripts as having been written by Galen, and Galen himself admits to having produced a work on this subject, is sufficient to outweigh them.

The position, however, is complicated by the fact that there is preserved in Istanbul the Arabic text of a different tract entitled Galen's Book on Regimen in Acute Diseases in accordance with the

---

[1] XIX 31,13 sq. & 36,17 sq. K. = Scr. min. II 109,21 & 113,19 sq.

[2] *Kitāb al-fihrist*, ed. Flügel (Leipzig 1871), vol. 1 p. 290.

[3] *Kitāb ʿuyūn al-anbāʾ*, ed. Müller (Cairo 1882), vol. 1 p. 98.

[4] *Taʾrīkh al-ḥukamāʾ*, ed. Lippert (Leipzig 1903), p. 131.

[5] Abhandlungen für die Kunde des Morgenlandes 17, 2 no. 78. It may be noted that the title of the work is given in a different form in Recension B of this work (Bergsträßer, Neue Materialien zu Ḥunain ibn Isḥāq's Galen-Bibliographie, Abhandlungen für die Kunde des Morgenlandes 19, 2 p. 47), where it is quoted as: *Tadbīr Abuqrāṭ li-l-amrāḍ al-ḥādda.*

[6] CMG V 9, 1.

Opinion of Hippocrates. The work is addressed to one Victorinus, who had asked the author for information on the specific point of whether or not Hippocrates used to allow food to patients suffering from acute diseases. There are a number of unflattering references to a previous informant of Victorinus, who had claimed that Hippocrates did not use a restrictive diet, and this view is refuted by reference to the following Hippocratic quotations, around which the text is constructed:

Aphor. I 8 (IV 464, 1 sq. L.) *ὁκόταν δὲ ἀκμάζῃ κτλ.*

De diaet. in morb. acut. I 128, 19–129, 2 Kw. *τοῦτο οὖν ἡγεῦμαι κτλ.*

ibid. 121, 16–20 *φημὶ γὰρ ἄμεινον κτλ.*

ibid. 118, 14–17 *ἔπειτα, ἢν μὲν ἄλγημα κτλ.*

ibid. 114, 13–16 *πλῆθος δὲ ἀρκεῖ κτλ.*

Aphor. I 10 (IV 464, 7–9 L.) *ὁκόσοισι μὲν οὖν κτλ.*

De diaet. in morb. acut. I 118, 3–6 Kw. *μάλα μὲν οὖν τὰ πλεῖστα κτλ.*

ibid. 137, 3–5 *ἄνευ μὲν ῥυφημάτων κτλ.*

ibid. 140, 6–8 *τοῖσι δὲ ποτῷ κτλ.*

ibid. 144, 21–145, 2 *χρῆσθαι δὲ λουτροῖσι κτλ.*

ibid. 122, 2–6 *οἶδα δὲ τοὺς ἰητροὺς κτλ.*

ibid. 129, 13–22 *πάντα οὖν ταῦτα κτλ.*

ibid. 133, 21–134, 2 *ἔπειτα οὐ χρηστέον ῥυφήμασιν κτλ.*

ibid. 127, 19–21 *τὴν ἀφαίρεσιν ὅλως ἀφελεῖν κτλ.*

Aphor. I 7 (IV 462, 12 sq. L.) *ὅκου μὲν κάτοξυ τὸ νούσημα κτλ.*

De diaet. in morb. acut. I 113, 19–114, 5 Kw. *πτισάνη μὲν οὖν δοκεῖ κτλ.*

It is clear from the introductory address as well as from these quotations, and, in fact, from the general style[1] and content of the work as a whole, that this text must be taken as reproducing a Greek original and cannot be dismissed as an Arab forgery. The Victorinus for whom it was written may perhaps be identified as C. Aufidius Victorinus, a friend of Marcus Aurelius and prefect of Rome under Commodus. In turn, he may reasonably be assumed to be the same man as "Victor, the eparch of Rome", mentioned in Galen's expanded commentary on Hippocrates' De diaeta in morbis acutis[2]. In this commentary, whose authenticity is unchallenged, Galen mentions a tract On Hippocrates' Regimen composed for this man by an unnamed doctor[3],

---

[1] As a particular instance of this may be noted a device foreign to Arab authors, the rhetorical praeteritio, p. 90,16 sqq.

[2] CMG V 9, 1 p. 265, 22. See also H. Pflaum, C. Aufidius Victorinus, Paris 1956.

[3] loc. cit.

whom he criticises for having distorted the following Hippocratic quotations:

a) De diaet. in morb. acut. I. 144, 20sq. Kw. *τοὺς δὲ φιλολουτρέοντας, οὐδ' εἰ δὶς τῆς ἡμέρης λούοις, οὐδὲν ἂν βλάπτοις*
b) ibid. p. 128, 20sq. *οὐ στερητέαι αἱ πρῶται ἡμέραι τοῦ ῥυφήματος*
c) ibid. p. 114, 9sq. *τοῖσι μέν γε εἰθισμένοισι δὶς σιτεῖσθαι τῆς ἡμέρης δὶς δοτέον*

Of these last two quotations Galen claims that the author of the tract has omitted half. They are thus presumably transformed into statements that patients suffering from acute diseases should always be fed, by the omission of the conclusion of (b), which runs: *τοῖσι μέλλουσιν ὀλίγον ὕστερον ῥυφήμασιν ἢ σιτίοισι χρῆσθαι* and by the omission, perhaps, of the words, *τοῖσι μέν γε εἰθισμένοισι δὶς σιτεῖσθαι* from (c).

The Arabic text also is concerned with criticism of the man who had told Victorinus that Hippocrates used to feed each day those suffering from acute diseases. The author notes: "He then betakes himself to words of Hippocrates which he produces for you in order to prove the truth of what he has to say. He divorces some of them from the context which gives them their full meaning; from some he leaves out what is necessary to complete the sense; another phrase he alters and he cuts the beginning from another."[1]

It is clear, then, that the Arabic reproduces the commentary's criticisms so exactly that it seems difficult to doubt that the same man was responsible for both. Other instances of marked similarity between the Arabic and the Greek of the commentary are listed in the notes on the translation. To these may be added more general indications of tone and matter. The references to Victorinus' unnamed informant show all Galen's characteristic intolerance of fools and charlatans, and the repetitive nature of the instruction fits in well with his expressed approval of Hippocrates' habit of repetition where the points involved are important[2]. Together with this may be noted a liking for textual excursus and grammatical discussion, as shown in the account of Hippocrates' phrase: Aphor. I 7 (IV 462, 13 L.) *τῇ ἐσχάτως λεπτοτάτῃ*[3],

---

[1] p. 106,11–13.
[2] In Hipp. De officina medici comm. XVIII B p. 884 K.
[3] p. 102,17f.

and in the textual variant noted in the phrase: De diaet. in morb. acut. I 118, 16sq. Kw. *μετὰ δὲ τὴν ἑβδόμην κτλ*[1].

As it stands, then, the Arabic provides a text which bears so close a relationship to Galen's style that, if it is not genuine, it must represent a conscious Greek forgery, for whose production it would seem hard to advance any plausible motive. It must therefore deserve serious consideration as being the text to which Galen refers in his De libris propriis. Had Westenberger's text been beyond suspicion, the assumption must have been that Galen composed two such works. As it stands, though, Westenberger's arguments in favour of the authenticity of his Greek text, derived as they are from Galen's references to his writings on this subject, can be used in their turn to support the Arabic and what Westenberger admits as legitimate doubts about the style and content of the Greek are then left unanswered. In view of this the claim must be advanced here that it is the Arabic and not the Greek that has preserved the authentic text of Galen.

The Arabic text is preserved in two Istanbul manuscripts, Aya Sofya 3631 (65^a–74^a) and Aya Sofya 3590 (75^a–88^a), noted by Ritter and Walzer in their article "Arabische Übersetzungen griechischer Ärzte in Stambuler Bibliotheken"[2]. Of these two manuscripts, Aya Sofya 3631 was fully described by Bergsträßer in the preface to his edition of Ḥunain's *Risāla*[3]. He notes of it that, though it is undated, it can be ascribed to the 7/8th century of the *Hijra*, that is to say the 13/14th centuries of the Christian era. Of Aya Sofya 3590, Ritter and Walzer state that it comes from a Spanish Arabic source and can be ascribed to the 6th century of the *Hijra*, that is to say the 12th century A. D. Aya Sofya 3631 is referred to here and throughout the Apparatus Criticus as A, while Aya Sofya 3590 is referred to as B. Both A and B share a number of common mistakes[4], but on the whole A gives the better text. It is not without instances of carelessness and its copyist may conceivably have been too cautious in other cases, but normally in the present edition its readings have been preferred to those of B in disputed passages. B serves to clear up a number of A's errors and, on occasions, its readings find support

---

1 p. 88,2.

2 Sitzungsber. d. Preuß. Akad. d. Wissensch., phil.-hist. Klasse, 1934, p. 815, no. 24.

3 op. cit., p. Isq.

4 For instance, they share the false reading الا الخطاء p. 106,17.

in the Arabic text of Hippocrates' De diaeta in morbis acutis[1]. It seems, however, to have been copied carelessly and it has a very large number of mistakes of omission as well as bad readings.

Bibliographical evidence, supported by that of the copyist of manuscript A, names the translator of this tract by Galen as Ḥunain ibn Isḥāq. In view of this, of Ḥunain's own remark, already quoted, and of the generally high standard of its Arabic style there seem on the face of it no reasonable grounds for doubting the ascription.

There is, however, some further evidence available that tends to complicate the position. In the first place, the exact relationship between the Arabic text of the quotations in this work and in the translation of Hippocrates is open to doubt. Further, Aya Sofya 3631 has preserved an epitome of this tract, attributed to Thābit ibn Qurra[2]. Perhaps the most remarkable thing about this is that, though there is no reason to doubt that Thābit knew of Hippocrates' text and of its lengthy commentary by Galen, he yet chose to epitomise a minor work dealing with one isolated problem that it presents. Apart from this, though, it must be asked whether in this epitome, which can be presumed to postdate the translation of the work itself, he made use of the text as it is presented here. The answer is not entirely clear. In the first place, his own mastery of Greek is undisputed and he could clearly have used the Greek original had it been available to him. Secondly, his technique of abridgement is such that he offers few occasions for direct comparison. What can be said is that the technicalities of his vocabulary are those of the present text, though this need not imply direct borrowing. In one passage, however, he keeps close enough to Hippocrates to be worth quoting in full. At the same time it is proposed to list the full tally of Hippocratic quotations. They are as follows:

I.

كشك الشعير عندى بالصواب اختير	كشك الشعير عندى بالصواب اختير
على سائر الاغذية التى تتخذ من الحبوب	على سائر الاغذية التى تتخذ من الحبوب
فى هذه الامراض واحمد من قدمه	فى هذه الامراض واحمد من لا يذمه
واختاره على غيره وذلك لان فيه لزوجة	واختاره على غيره وذلك لان فيه لزوجة

[1] Cambridge Middle East Centre, Arabic Technical and Scientific Texts, vol. 1 Heffer, 1966.

[2] Ritter & Walzer, op. cit., p. 832.

معها ملاسة واتصال ولين وزلق ورطوبة
معتدلة وتسكين للعطش وسرعة انغسال
ان احتيج الى ذلك ايضا منه وليس
فيه قبض ولا تهييج ردىء ولا ينتفخ
ويربو فى المعدة لانه قد انتفخ وربا
فى الطبخ غاية ما كان يمكن فيه ان
ينتفخ ويربو

Hippocrates I 113, 19–114, 5 Kw.

معها ملاسة واتصال ولين وزلق ورطوبة
معتدلة وتسكين للعطش وسرعة انغسال
ان احتيج الى ذلك ايضا منه وليس
فيه قبض ولا تهيّج ردىء ولا ينتفخ
ويربو فى المعدة لانه قد انتفخ وربا
فى الطبخ غاية ما كان يمكن فيه ان
ينتفخ ويربو

Galen p. 108, 18–110, 6

انما اختار ابقراط من الاحساء مـاء الشعير لانه احمد من غيره اذ كانت فيه ازوجة وملاسة واتصال ولين وزلق ورطوبة وتسكين للعطش وان الشىء الذى يتعلق منه بالحلق والمرىء ان احتاج الانسان ان يغسله ببعض الاشربة انغسل ولم يتعلق تعلقا شديدا مثل غيره من الاحساء التى يقف منها الشىء بعد الشىء وتجففه حرارة الحمى على الموضع فيعسر تبرئته منه وليس يهيج الوجع لكن يسكنه ولا ينتفخ ويربوا ، فى المعدة لانه قد انتفخ وربا فى الطبخ غاية ما يمكن فيه

Thābit ibn Qurra, Aya Sofya 3631: 46b l.12 sqq.

II.

ينبغى ان يعطى المريض فى اول الامر
مقدارا ليس بالكثير ولا بالغليظ لاكن
كيما يكون قد ورد البدن شىء بسبب
العادة ولا يفرط فيه خلاء العروق

Hippocrates I 114, 13–16 Kw.

يكتفى ان يعطى المريض فى اول مرضه
مقدارا ليس بالكثير ولا بالغليظ لكن
كيما يكون قد ورد البدن شىء بسبب
العادة ولا يفرط فيه خلاء العروق

Galen p. 88, 19 sq.

III.

طريق الرفد فى اكثر الامر طريق واحد
لمن يستعمل ماء الشعير ومعه ثفله ولمن
يستعمل مـاءه فقط ولمن لا يستعمل
واحـدا منهمـا لكن يقتصر على مـا

طريق الرفد فى اكثر الامر طريق واحد
لمن يستعمل ماء الشعير ومعه ثفله ولمن
يستعمل ماءه فقط ولمن لا يستعمل
واحدا منهما بتة لكن يقتصر على ما

---

1 *sic*

2 Galen, On the parts of medicine

يشرب وربما كان طريق الرفد مختلفا	يشرب وربما كان طريق الرفد مختلفا
Hippocrates I 118, 3–6 Kw.	Galen p. 94, 6–9

IV.

فانه ان كان فى الموضع وجع او رايت بالعليل احد الاعراض التى يتخوف منها عليه فينبغى ان يكون ما تعطيه من الحساء مقدارا ليس بالغليظ ولا بالكثير ويكون اعطاؤك اياه بعد اليوم السابع ان كانت قوته محتملة	ثم من بعد ان كان يجد المريض وجعا او ظهر فيه شىء من الاعراض المخوفة فينبغى ان يعطى الحسو وهو ليس بالغليظ ولا بالكثير من بعد اليوم السابع ان كان قويا
Hippocrates I 118, 14–17 Kw.	Galen p. 86, 19–88, 2

V.

فانى اقول ان ابتداء تناول المريض للحسو منذ اول الامر اجود من ان يسبق فيستعمل خلاء العروق ثم يبتدئ بتناول الحسو فى اليوم الثالث من مرضه او فى الرابع او فى الخامس او فى السادس او فى السابع الا ان يتقدم بحران المريض فيكون فى هذه المدة	فانى اقول ان ابتداء بتناول المريض للحسو منذ اول الامر اجود من ان يسبق فيستعمل خلاء العروق ثم يبتدئ بتناول الحسو فى اليوم الثالث من مرضه او فى الرابع او فى الخامس او فى السادس او فى السابع الا ان يتقدم بحران المرض فيكون فى هذه المدة
Hippocrates I 121, 16–20 Kw.	Galen p. 84, 20–23

VI.

وقد اعرف كثيرا من الاطباء يفعل ضد ما ينبغى ان يفعل وذلك انهم كلهم يجففون المرضى منذ اول المرض بيومين او ثلاثة او اكثر ثم ينيلونهم الاحساء والاشربة	وقد اعرف كثيرا من الاطباء يفعل ضد ما ينبغى ان يفعل وذلك انهم كلهم يجففون ابدان المرضى منذ اول المرض يومين او ثلاثة او اكثر من ذلك ثم ينيلونهم الاحساء والاشربة
Hippocrates I 122, 2–6 Kw.	Galen p. 96, 12–14

VII.

وقد ينبغى فى مواضع كثيرة ان يدفع الغذاء بتة وذلك متى كان المريض يحتمل ان يبقى الى ان يبلغ مرضه منتهاه وينضج

Galen p. 100, 5–7

وذلك ان النقصان فى الجملة انفع فى اكثر الامر متى كان المريض محتملا ما دام مرضه واقفا الى ان يبلغ منتهاه وينضج

Hippocrates I 127, 19–21 Kw.

VIII.

من اعظم جميع ما افيدكه عندى نفعا انه لا ينبغى ان تمنع المريض فى الايام الاول من مرضه ثم من بعد الاحساء على انها تختلف وانت مزمع بعد قليل ان تغذوه ببعض تلك الاحساء

Galen p. 82, 13–16

من اعظم ما افيدكه نفعا انه لا ينبغى ان تمنع المريض فى الايام الاول من مرضه بعض الاحساء على انها تختلف وانت مزمع بعد قليل ان تغذوه ببعض تلك الاحساء

Hippocrates I 128, 19–129, 2 Kw.

IX.

ففى جميع هذه الاشياء التى وصفت اعظم الدلائل على ان تدبير هولاء الاطباء للمرضى ليس بصواب لكنهم يستعملون خلاء العروق فى امراض لا ينبغى استعماله فيها وهم سيغذون اصحابها بعد بالاحساء ويغيرون التدبير وينقلونه [1] من خلاء العروق الى استعمال الاحساء فى امراض لا ينبغى ان يغير فيها وهم فى اكثر الامر من ذلك على خطاء وذلك انهم كانوا كثيرا ما ينقلون المريض من خلاء العروق الى استعمال الاحساء فى الاوقات التى

(ففى ——— يغير فيها desunt in codd.)

وهم فى اكثر الامر من ذلك على خطاء وذلك انهم كثيرا ما ينقلون المريض من خلاء العروق الى استعمال الاحساء فى الاوقات التى

[1] فينقلونه p. 98 l. 1

ينتفع فيها كثيرا بالنقلة من الاحساء
الى المشارفة لخلاء العروق ان اتفق ان
يكون استصعاب المرض فى ذلك الوقت

Galen p. 100, 19–102, 4
(cf. p. 96, 20–98, 2)

ينتفع فيها كثيرا بالنقلة من الاحساء الى
استعمال خلاء العروق ان اتفق ان
يكون استصعاب المرض فى ذلك الوقت

Hippocrates I 129, 13–22 Kw.

X.

ثم من بعد فلا ينبغى ان تستعمل
الاحساء دون ان ينضج المرض او تظهر
علامة اخرى فى الامعاء تدل على خلاء
العروق او على شىء مهيج

Galen p. 98, 9 sq. 17 sq.
(cf. p. 100, 10 sq.)

ثم لا يستعمل بعده شىء من الاحساء
دون ان ينضج المرض او تظهر فى
الامعاء علامة اخرى تدعو الى ترك المنع
من استعمال الغذاء او علامة مهيجة

Hippocrates I 133, 21–134,2 Kw.

XI.

وان تجنبت الاحساء واقتصرت على
ماء العسل فى هذه الامراض كان
صوابك كثيرا وخطاؤك قليلا غير كثير

Galen p. 94, 9–11

اذا استعملت فى هذه الامراض مكان
الاحساء وكل ما يشرب ماء العسل
كان صوابا فى اشياء كثيرة ولم يمكن ان
تخطئ كثير خطاء

Hippocrates I 137, 3–5 Kw.

XII.

فاما من يقتصر على التدبير بما يشرب
فقط من غير ان يرزأ شيئا من الاحساء
فلهذا السبب لا يوافقه ان يقتصر على
ذلك دائما

Galen p. 94, 13–16

فاما من يستعمل فى تدبيره ما يشرب
فقط ولا يتناول كشك الشعير فليس
يوافقه استعمال السكنجبين وحده

Hippocrates I 140, 6–8 Kw.

XIII.

استعمال الاستحمام فى الحمام لمن
يستعمل ماء الشعير مع ثفله امكن منه
لمن يقتصر على مائه وقد يقدر من يقتصر
على ماء الشعير كثيرا على استعمال

استعمال الاستحمام فيمن يتناول كشك
الشعير ومعه ثفله امكن منه كثيرا فيمن
يستعمل ماءه فقط وربما امكن استعمال
الاستحمام فى هؤلاء ايضا واقل ما

يمكن استعماله فيمن كان يتدبر بالاشربة فقط	الحمام فاما من يقتصر على ما يشرب فقط فلا يكاد يقدر على استعمال الحمام
Hippocrates I 144, 21–145, 2 Kw.	Galen p. 94, 13–16

The evidence of this list may not be conclusive, but it is at least suggestive. The similarity between the text of the passage quoted from Thābit's epitome and those of the other two works is probably enough to indicate that Thābit knew of both, or at least of one of them, and was prepared to follow their lead. If this is accepted, though, it must be noted that he was willing to go to considerable lengths to expand and explain the term *εὐέκπλυτον* translated in the other two works by سرعة انغسال.

The relationship between the Arabic text of Hippocrates and of Galen is more doubtful. It seems impossible to explain their similarities as coincidental in view not only of the lengths of the passages involved but also of the shared oddities of some of the Arabic translations[1]. This problem was discussed in the Introduction to the published text of the Arabic translation of the Hippocratic original. A tentative solution was put forward to the effect that the Arabic represents a version made by ʿĪsā ibn Yaḥyā based on a Syrian translation by Ḥunain. Ḥunain, it was suggested, might reasonably be supposed to have used this in preparing the present work, changing it where he thought fit. This, though plainly a matter of conjecture and not of proof, would at least reconcile the evidence as it stands and it would serve to confirm the attribution of the present translation to Ḥunain, an attribution which it is proposed here to accept.

My thanks are due to Dr. Kollesch and to Dr. Strohmaier for the help and advice that they have given me in the preparation of these editions. In particular, I am indebted to Dr. Strohmaier for a number of corrections, over and above the suggestions which he has made and which are recorded in the Apparatus.

Cambridge, October 1966 Malcolm Lyons

[1] As an instance may be quoted the unusual translation of the phrase *τοῦτο οὖν ἡγεῦμαι μέγιστον διδακτήϱιον* (I 128, 19 Kw.); cf. p. 19 l. 8.

CONSPECTVS SIGLORVM

Ms. = Aya Sofya 3725
S' = correctiones primae manus

مقالة جالينوس فى أجزاء الطبّ

GALEN'S TREATISE ON THE PARTS OF MEDICINE

مقالة جالينوس فى أجزاء الطبّ

١ قال جالينوس أظنّ بك يا حبيبى ايوسطس أن بالواجب تحيّرت فى أمر
٢ أجزاء الطبّ لأنّ القدماء قد اختلفوا فى قسمتها فترى بعضهم قد قسم صناعة
الطبّ كلّها إلى علاج اليد واستعمال الأدوية والتدبير ثمّ أنّهم بعد قسموا كلّ
واحد من هذه الأجزاء ليس على مثال واحد وبعضهم قسموا الطبّ قسمين أحدهما
الشفاء والآخر حفظ الصحّة وقوم رأوا أنّه ينبغى أن يضاف إلى هذه قسم آخر
وهو التقدّم فى حفظ الصحّة وقوم آخرون رأوا أنّه ينبغى أن يضاف إلى هذه
قسم آخر وهو تلافى الصحّة وبعضهم رأى أنّه ينبغى أن يضاف إليهما الجزآن
٣ جميعا ويضاف إليهما جزء آخر وهو حفظ خصب البدن وقد أضاف قوم إلى
هذه الأجزاء تدبير المشائخ لأنّه جزء خاصّ من صناعة الطبّ وبعضهم أضاف إلى
ذلك مع تدبير المشائخ تدبير الصبيان وأضاف قوم آخرون إلى هذه التزيّن الطبّىّ
٤ وفرقوا بينه وبين التزيّن للتحسين وقد قصد قوم لتكثير أجزاء الطبّ بأكثر ممّا
كثّروها هؤلاء فأضافوا إلى هذه الأجزاء التى ذكرنا جزءا آخر صغيرا منذ أوّل القسمة
وهو رياضة الصوت ومنهم من أضاف هذا على الإطلاق وعلى غير تمييز وبعضهم
ميّز فبيّن أنّ بعض من يقصد لتخريج الصوت يصلح لمن يناضل فى الصوت
أعنى من يروم أن يغالب غيره فيه وبعضهم إنّما يقصد لأن يكون الصوت فيه
٥ باقيا على طبيعته كسائر الأفعال الأخر إلّا أنّه قد يجب على هؤلاء أن يقيموا لكلّ
واحد من الأفعال الجزئيّة التى فى البدن جزءا خاصّا من هذه الصناعة ولو كانوا
فعلوا ذلك لكانت قسمتهم واجبة لكنّهم لمّا أغفلوا الأفعال الباقية فيه

1 *ante titulum add.* بسم الله الرحمن الرحيم Ms.   6 قسما Ms.   8 قسما Ms.   إليهما *sic*   الجزئين Ms.

GALEN'S TREATISE ON THE PARTS OF MEDICINE

1. Galen said: My dear Justus, I think that you have good reason
to be confused on the subject of the parts of medicine. For *the ancients*[1] 2
differed in their division in that some of them, as you see, divided all
medicine into *surgery, pharmacy* and diet, and then afterwards they
subdivided each of these parts, but not *in the same way*. Others amongst
them divided it in two, one section being the therapeutic and the other
dealing with the preservation of health. Here some hold that one
should add another section, the prophylactic, and others another, the
recuperative, while there are those who think that both of these should
be added to the first two sections and another put in as well, namely
that which preserves eutrophy. *To these divisions* geriatrics has been 3
added as being a special branch of medicine and this has been coupled
by some with paediatrics. Others have added to these the art of cosmetics, used medicinally, as distinguished from its use in beauty-treatment.

A number have tried to multiply the parts of medicine even more 4
than this. To what we have already mentioned they have added another small primary division, which is that of speech training. This
has been put in by some absolutely and without distinction, whereas
others have made a distinction and have shown that *attempts at voice
production may be suitable from the point of view of competition – that
is for those who wish to surpass others in this* – whereas in other cases
the object is simply to ensure that the voice remains in its natural
state, this being on a par with the position in respect of all our other
actions. These people, however, must then assign to each one of the 5
actions of parts in the body a special branch of medicine and were
they, in fact, to do that, then their division would be logically sound.
However, they have ignored all other physical actions and mentioned

[1] Italics in the text of Galen indicate that the passage is found in a different form in the Latin version.

كلّها وذكروا فعلا واحدا كشفوا من خطاء أنفسهم أنّ قسمتهم غير محكمة ولا واجبة ولا الذين قسموا الطبّ إلى أعظم أجزائه بمتّفقين فى قسمة تلك الأجزاء إلى الأجزاء التى هى أصغر منها وقد عمد قوم إلى بعض تلك الأجزاء فوضعوها ٦ أجزاء للطبّ ونقصوا أجزاء كثيرة منها وأضافوا إليها أجزاء أخر فى القسمة الأولى مثل الكلام فى الأمور الطبيعيّة والكلام فى العلل   قال حنين يعنى بالكلام فى العلل معرفة الأمراض   وقد أضاف قوم إلى هذه جزءا آخر سمّوه الموادّىّ

أىّ الأجزاء يعنى الموادّىّ سيشرح جالينوس فيما بعد

وأضاف إليه آخرون استخراج الدلائل وأضاف إليه آخرون الكلام فى الأسباب

٢ وأمّا أصحاب التجارب فكلّهم إلاّ الشاذّ منهم متّفقون على أنّ فصول الطبّ الأول الجنسيّة فصلان وذلك أنّهم قالوا انّ منها أجزاء متمّمة ومنها أجزاء مقوّمة ولم يوافق بعضهم بعضا فى إحصاء هذه الأجزاء وذلك أنّ بعضهم قال انّ الأجزاء المتمّمة للطبّ هى الاستدلال والشفاء وقد عدّ قوم مع هذه حفظ الصحّة وأضاف إلى هذه معها قوم التزيين الطبّىّ وبعضهم أضاف إليها رياضة الصوت وأمّا الأجزاء المقوّمة للطبّ فجعلوها كلّهم العيان والخبر وقوم منهم لا كلّهم عدّوا النقلة من الشىء إلى نظيره جزءا من صناعة الطبّ وليس يوافق جميع ٢ أصحاب التجارب وأصحاب الرأى بعضهم بعضا فى قسمة كلّ واحد من هذه ‹ إلى › الأجزاء التى هى أصغر منها لا أهل إحدى الفرقتين ولا أهل الفرقة الواحدة الأخرى   قال حنين إحدى الفرقتين يعنى به فرقة أصحاب التجارب وفرقة أصحاب الرأى إذ كانت أهل فرقة أصحاب التجارب ليس يوافق بعضهم بعضا وكذلك فرقة أصحاب الرأى ويعنى بالفرقة الواحدة الأخرى أهل فرقة أصحاب التجارب لا أهل فرقة الرأى   وإن عدّ عادّ هذه النتف الصغار الكثيرة أجزاء من صناعة الطبّ على ما قد يتّسم الآن برومية خاصّة حتّى يسمّوا بعض الأطبّاء معالجى الأسنان ويسمّوا بعضهم معالجى الآذان ويسمّوا بعضهم معالجى المقعدة أفضى القول إلى حيرة أعظم من هذه على أنّ أصحاب هذا الشأن أيضا قد وجدوا فرصة من اسم قد وضع لا منذ قريب

5 الطبيعة Ms.   14 كلها Ms.: *sec. Lat. correxi*   17 إلى *sec. Lat. supplevi*

one only, thus showing themselves to be at fault in having made an unsound and illogical division. As for those who have divided medicine into its main sections, they are not agreed in their subdivisions. Some 6
of these have been taken and posited as parts of the art of medicine. Many have been dropped while others have been added in the primary division. Examples of these latter are physiology and pathology. – *Ḥunain said: By "pathology" he means the knowledge of diseases.* – To these some have added another branch which they have called "the material" – *Which part is meant by "the material" will be explained by Galen later*[1]. –, while others have added the diagnostic section and others aetiology.

2. The Empiricists, with a few exceptions, are agreed that the prime generic divisions of medicine are two in number, in that they say that some of its parts are perfective and others constitutive, though they are not agreed about their numbering. Some of them have stated the perfective parts to be the diagnostic and the therapeutic, to which have been added by different authorities sections dealing with the preservation of health, the medical use of cosmetics, and speech training. As for the constitutive parts, they have all taken these to be observation and information, while some, though not all, have taken the switch from one thing to what is like it (differential diagnosis) to be a part of the art of medicine.

In the splitting of each of these sections into its subdivisions there 2
is no general agreement amongst the Empiricists or the Dogmatists, between the members of the one school or of the other. – *Ḥunain said: When he says "the one school" he refers to the Empiricists and the Dogmatists, since there was no internal agreement amongst either the former or the latter. When he says "the other" he means the Empiricists and not the Dogmatists.* – So it may happen that these many small sections are counted parts of the art of medicine and it is in this way that one finds, particularly at Rome in these days, distinguishing titles by which some doctors are known as dentists, others as otologists and others as specialists in the posterior. This argument, however, leads to even greater mystification, although its protagonists can find an opportune defence provided them by a title that is not

---

[1] Ḥunain's name is not given here and this may be assumed to be a copyist's gloss.

لكن منذ مدّة من الزمان بعيدة جدّا وهى صناعة أصحاب علاج العين فإنّه إن كانت العينان مفردة بطبيب على حدته لما خرج من الواجب أن يكون للأسنان أيضا طبيب آخر مفرد على حدته وآخر للأذنين وآخرون لكلّ واحد من أعضاء البدن فيجب من ذلك أن يكون عدد الأطبّاء بعدد أعضاء البدن وإذ كان أيضا بعض الأطبّاء قد يسمّون قدّاحى الأعين وبعضهم بطّاطى القيل وبعضهم مخرجى الحصى وبعضهم على مثال آخر شبيه بهذا فقد يجب أن تصير عدّة الأطبّاء أكثر كثيرا من عدد أعضاء البدن وذلك أنّه ليس إنّما يوجد لكلّ واحد من الأعضاء طبيب مفرد على حدته فقط لكن قد يوجد لكلّ واحدة من علل كلّ واحد من الأعضاء طبيب مفرد على حدته وخليق ألاّ تكون تعجب أن تنقسم ٣
هذه الصناعة لعظمها فى المدينة العظيمة إلى هذه الأقسام التى هى بهذا العدد الكثير إذ كانت الصناعة لعظمها لا يمكن الأطبّاء كلّهم أن يستوعبوها عن آخرها وكانت هذه المدينة لعظمها يجد فيها جميعهم معاشا فإنّ المدينة الصغيرة لا يجد فيها معاشا من يقتدح الأعين ولا من يبطّ القيل فأمّا رومية واسكندريّة فلكثرة من بهما من الناس هما ملئان بأن يجد فيهما من يعالج جزءا واحدا من الطبّ معاشه فضلا عن من معه من الطبّ أكثر من ذلك فأمّا فى المدن الأخر الصغار فقد يضطرّ من كان إنّما يعالج من الطبّ فنّا واحدا أن ينتقل من مدينة إلى مدينة انتقالا متواترا حتّى يكون الشىء الذى هو لأهل ايطاليا برومية وحدها لأولائك مثلا بلد اليونانيّين كلّه

٣ وقد رأيت أنّه يحسن أن أبتدئ فى هذا الموضع بالمعنى الذى أقصد إليه إذ كان قد بان من أمر أجزاء هذه الصناعة التى هى أقلّ أجزائها كيف الحال فى طبيعتها وأن أتقدّم فألخّص تلخيصا بيّنا أىّ الأجزاء هى التى ينبغى أن تسمّى أقلّ الأجزاء بعد أن أضع لقولى مثالا ليس من شىء خارج عن الغرض الذى قصدت إليه لكن من شىء نافع فيه ومنفعته ليس بدون منفعة غيره فأقول انّه ٢
كما نقصد فى التشريح فى أجزاء البدن أن نبلغ أقصى ما يوجد منها فى القلّة فى الصورة وهى التى نسمّيها الأركان المحسوسة فنفهمها ونقف على حقائقها كذلك ينبغى أن نروم وجود أجزاء الطبّ كلّه حتّى نبلغ أقلّ قليل أجزائه فأقول انّ ٣

3 أعضاء *ex* الاعضاء *corr.* S[1] 14 ملئان *sic* 17 لأولئك Ms. 18 *fort.* ببلد *legendum est*

recent but is, rather, of very long standing, – I refer to the art of the oculist. For if the eyes have a specialist to deal with them, it is not unnatural to suppose that there should be a specialist for the teeth, another for the ears and others for each part of the body. It follows that there should be as many doctors as there are parts of the body. But one further finds that some doctors are known as couchers of cataracts and others as men who cut hernias or who remove stones and there are others who have different titles on the same pattern. So it follows that the number of doctors should very much exceed the number of these parts. For not only will there be a single specialist to deal with each part of the body individually, but each of the ailments of each of the parts will have its separate specialist.

You should not be surprised if the scope of the art of medicine 3
causes it to be divided in a great city into this large number of sections. *For thanks to its extent not all doctors can master it in its entirety and in this city, because of its size, all of them can find a living.* In a small town, of course, this is not possible for oculists and those who cut hernias. So as far as Rome and Alexandria are concerned, the number of their inhabitants ensures a livelihood for those who practise any single branch of medicine there, let alone those who have more medical competence than that. Elsewhere, however, where towns are small, the single branch specialists must travel continuously from place to place, so that all Greece, for instance, may provide for them what Rome by itself provides for the Italians[1].

3. I have thought it proper to start here by mentioning what I have in mind. The natural state of the minutest parts of the art of medicine has already been clearly shown. My first task, therefore, must be to produce a clear summary of which these parts are that should be called the smallest. First, however, I shall produce an example taken from something that is not extraneous to my present purpose but, rather, from what is useful to it – no less useful, in fact, than anything else of the kind.

I say that our object in the dissection of parts of the body is to 2
arrive at the smallest formations[2] found there, which we call "the sensible elements", and to reach an understanding of their real nature. Similarly we must try to find out in full the parts of the art of medicine

[1] I. e. the Italian specialists.

[2] Here εἶδος (lat. species) has been mistranslated by *ṣūra*.

أجزاء بدن الإنســان التى هى أعظم أجزائه هى الرأس والصدر والبطن واليدان قال حنين اليد يعنى بها كلّ ما هو من دون المنكب من العضد والساعد والكفّ والرجلان قال حنين الرجل يعنى بها كلّ ما هو من دون الورك من الفخذ والساق والقدم وأجزاء كلّ واحد من هذه أيضـا أمّا أجزاء الرأس فالجزء الـذى يخصّ بهذا الاسم أعنى الرأس والأذنان والوجه والرقبة وأمّا الجزء الذى يخصّ باسم الرأس وهو الجزء الذى الشعر فيه نابت من جملة الرأس فأجزاؤه الموجودة فى القسمة الأولى الدماغ والأمّان المحيطان به وقحف الرأس والعروق الضوارب وغير الضوارب والأغشية والأعصاب والجلد ولكلّ واحد من هذه الأجزاء أجزاء أخر أكثر منها وسنتكلّم فى جميعها فى كتاب علاج التشريح فأمّا فى هذا المذهب الذى نحن فيه فقد يكتفى أن نقصد إلى واحد منهـا دون غيره أىّ واحد كـان فيتبيّن فيه قسمة البدن حتّى ننتهى إلى الأركـان المحسوسة فأقول انّ العرق الضارب فى نفسه هو ذو طبقتين وإنّما قلت فى نفسه من قبل أنّى ٤ قد بيّنت فى غير هذا الموضع أنّه ربّما لحقه بسبب من الأسباب يعرض له أن يوجد إمّا ذو ثلث طبقات وإمّا ذو أربع طبقات وإحدى هاتين الطبقتين مؤلّفة من شظايا تمتدّ عرضا والطبقة الأخرى مؤلّفة من شظايا تمتدّ على الاستقامة طولا وليس تقدر أن تقسم هذه الشظايا إلى صورة أخرى بل هذا هو الجزء الذى لا يحتمل القسمة وهو أصغر الأجزاء فى الصورة ومن عادتنا أن نسمّى الأجزاء من ٥ البدن الموكّلة بفعل واحد من الأفعـال إمّا ضرورىّ لبـدن الحىّ بأسره وإمّا نافع له آلات وأمّا الأجزاء التى هـى أكبر من هذه فنسمّيها أجزاء فقط كما نسمّى الرأس بأسره وأمّا الأجزاء التى هى أصغر من تلك وهى متشابهة الأجزاء غير منقسمة فى الصورة فليس نقتصر على أن نسمّيها أجزاء فقط لكن نسمّيها أيضا الأركان المحسوسة من البدن والأركان المحسوسة هى الشظايا من كلّ واحدة من الآلات وغيرهـا من أشياء سأذكرها بعد فإنّ الشريانات والأعصاب والعروق والأمعاء والمعدة والرحم والمثانة كلّها على مثال واحد مركّبة أبدانها أعنى أجرامها من شظايا ومن أركان البدن المحسوسة معما ذكرت من الشظايا الأغشية أيضا والرباطات وهى العصب واللحم أعنى اللحم البسيط المفرد واللحم الخاصّ بكلّ واحد من الأحشاء

5 والجزء Ms. والأذنين Ms. 12 العرق *ex* العروق *corr.* S¹ 25 الشظايا الأغشية] الشظايا Ms. : فى أخرى الأغشية *in marg.* S¹ هى *deleverit* Strohmaier

until we arrive at its smallest components. I say, then, that the main 3
parts of the human body are the head, the chest, the belly, the hands – *Ḥunain said: By the term yad he means the whole of the upper arm, the fore-arm and the hand from the shoulder down.* –, the feet – *Ḥunain said: By the term riǧl he means the thigh, leg and foot from the hip down.* –, and next come the subdivisions of each of these. As for the parts of the head, *there is what is particularized by this term – that is, "head"* – together with the ears, the face and the neck. The primary divisions of what is specifically called "head", which is that part of the whole where the hair grows, are the brain, the dura and the pia mater, the skull, the arteries and veins, the membranes, nerves and skin. Each of these has a number of further subdivisions and *we shall discuss* them all in our work "On Anatomy". From the point of view of our present concerns it is enough for us to concentrate on one part, whichever this may be, to the exclusion of the others, and to show there how the body can be divided up until the *sensible* elements are reached.

I say, then, that the artery, in itself, has two tunics. – I have added 4
"in itself" because, as I have shown elsewhere, thanks to some adventitious cause you may happen to find it with either three or four tunics. – One of these two is composed of fibres stretched transversely while those of the other run lengthwise. The fibres cannot be subdivided into any other form[1] but, rather, they represent what is indivisible and most minute in form[1].

It is a habit of ours to use the term "organ" of those parts of the 5
body that are entrusted with the control of any single action that is either necessary or useful to the whole animal body. What are bigger than these we simply call parts, an example being the whole head, while what is smaller and is homoiomerous and not formally divisible is called a sensible element of the body and not just a part. These sensible elements are the fibres of each of the organs *as well as other things that I shall mention later*. For the arteries, *the nerves, the veins*, the intestines, the stomach, the womb and the bladder are all alike in that their *bodies, by which I mean their structures*, are compounded of fibres. In addition to these fibres that I have mentioned, the sensible elements are the membranes and the connective parts, that is the nerves and the flesh. By 'flesh' I mean, what is simply flesh and what is peculiar to the individual intestines and is known to some as "the

---

[1] Here εἶδος (lat. species) has been mistranslated by *ṣūra*.

الذى لقّبه قوم بالحشو ومع تلك الأجزاء أيضا العظام والغضاريف والسمين وسائر
ما هو على هذا المثال فبالواجب يسمّى المسمّى هذه أركانا محسوسة لأبداننا وأمّا ٦
الجنس الآخر من الأجزاء الذى هو آلىّ فما بأس بذكر هذا أيضا فهو العروق
الضوارب وغير الضوارب والأعصاب والكلى والمعدة والطحال والكبد والرئة والقلب
وما كان من غير ذلك على هذا المثال

٤ وعلى قياس هذا المثال فينبغى أن نتوهّم على صناعة القدح للماء فى العين
أنّها إنّما هى جزء من صناعة الطبّ كلّها على مثال ما هو جزء من بدن الإنسان
كلّه العضو الذى يسمّى آلة من الآلات وكلّ واحد من أجزاء صناعة قدح الماء الذى
فى العين نظير الأركان المحسوسة من البدن وأجزاء هذه الصناعة هى العلوم التى فى النفس ٢
منّا وهى التى تسمّى أبواب العلم أوّلها علم جملة صورة المقداح والثانى معرفة الجزء
من العين الذى ينبغى يقتدح فيه والثالث معرفة تقدير تعويضه قال حنين
يعنى نحو الحدقة والرابع معرفة تقدير إحالته والخامس معرفة تقدير الماء ونقله
من الموضع الذى يثبت فيه قال حنين يعنى الحدقة والسادس
معرفة تقدير إبعاده والسابع معرفة تقدير تغليقه فإنّ هذه الأجزاء هى أقصى العلوم
وأقلّ قليلها وأبسطها وما لا يقبل منها القسمة إلى علوم أخر هى أبسط منها وعلوما
قلت أو معارف أو حكما أو أبواب علم فلا تتوهّمنّ أن بين قولى فى هذا فرق أصلا
فى هذا الفنّ الذى قصدنا إليه وكذلك أجزاء قلت أو أعضاء أو نتفا فلا فرق بين
ذلك فى هذا الفنّ فعلم القدح مركّب من هذه العلوم الجزئيّة التى عددت وأمّا ٣
جملة شفاء الماء المتولّد فى العين فيحتاج مع هذه الى علمين آخرين أحدهما متقدّم
فى مرتبته وهو الذى يتقدّم فيهيّئ والآخر هو الذى به يتمّ الشفاء فإنّ الطبيب إذا ٤
تضمّن علاج من به ماء فى عينيه وكان فى بدنه امتلاء كبير أعنى كثرة من الأخلاط
أو خلط ردىء أو صداع فرام قبل أن يصلح من هذه الأشياء أن يعالج عينه بالقدح

11 تغويصه *legerit* Strohmaier 14 تعليقه Ms. 16 معارفا Ms.

stuffing"[1]. In addition to these parts there are the bones, the carti-
lages, the fat and other similar things and these are rightly called the
sensible elements of our bodies. Nor is there any harm in our mentioning 6
the other class of parts as well, that is, the organic. For this class is
composed of the *arteries and veins*, the nerves, the kidneys, the
stomach, the spleen, the liver, the lungs, the heart and other similar
parts.

4. On this analogy, then, we should assume of the art of couching
cataracts that it is a part of the whole art of medicine in the same way
that the member which we call an organ is part of the whole human
body and each of the parts of cataract couching is the equivalent of a
sensible element of the body. They represent, in fact, the facets of 2
knowledge that we have and they are what are called "the gates of
knowledge". First comes the knowledge of the whole form *of the
couching needle;* second, that of the part of the eye where the cataract
must be treated; third, that of the proper measurement involved in
its *replacement* – *Ḥunain said: He means "towards the pupil"*. –;
fourth, that of the proper measurements involved in its conversion;
fifth, that of those relating to the cataract and its shifting from the
place of its lodgement – *Ḥunain said: He means the pupil.*–; sixth,
that of those relating to its removal and seventh, that of those involved
in its closure. These, then, are the ultimate, the most minute and the
simplest of the sciences, which accept no division into others simpler
than themselves. Incidentally, whether I talk of sciences, branches of
knowledge or of wisdom, or gates of knowledge, you should not
imagine that any difference is implied as far as this field is concerned
with which we are dealing. Similarly, if I talk of parts, members, or
particles, no difference is meant here.

The science of couching cataracts, is compounded of these partial 3
branches of knowledge that I have numbered, but for the full cure of
the fluid generated in the eye you need *two more in addition to them.*
Of these two, one is preliminary and it is this that first prepares the
ground, while the other provides the completion of the cure. It may be, 4
then, that a doctor has to undertake the treatment of a cataract
patient who is suffering from a form of plethory – I mean a quantity
of humours – or from an evil humour or from a headache. If he sets
about couching the cataract before these things are put right, he will

---

[1] *παρέγχυμα.*

3 Galen, On the parts of medicine

أحدث ورما فى الطبقات التى ينقبها و يكسب للرأس كلّه مشاركة فى العلّة للعين فكى
لا يكون ذلك يحتاج إلى الصناعة التى تتقدّم فتعدّ وتهيّئ والغرض فيها أن ينقى جملة
البدن من الفضل ويسكّن الوجع عن الرأس والعلوم التى منها تكون هذه الأشياء هى
أركان صناعة الطبّ وكذلك أيضا العلوم التى منها من بعد القدح نحفظ العينين حتّى
لا يحدث فيها ورم ونحفظ الرأس حتّى لا يحدث فيه وجع هى أركان من أركان الطبّ
أعنى أجزاء من أقصى أجزائه وما لا يكون أقلّ منه وينبغى أن ينقل هذا القول الذى ٥
أجريته على طريق المثال إلى جميع العلل حتّى يكون علم شفاء كلّ واحد منها أىّ
علّة كانت جزءا من الطبّ نظير لما هو جزء من بدن الحيوان ذلك الجزء الذى
يسمّى آلة من الآلات وهاهنا أيضا موضع غلط قبل أن نلخّص جملة هذا
المعنى حتّى نستقصى تلخيصها فإنّ ظانّا لعلّه يظنّ أنّه كما أنّ للماء فى العين
صناعة تشفيه كذلك للورم على الإطلاق قال حنين افهم من قوله
فى هذا الموضع الورم الذى يحدث عن الدم الذى يسمّيه اليونانيّون فلغمونى فإنّ
هذا وحده يسمّونه ورما على الإطلاق صناعة تشفيه وعلى هذا المثال
للقرحة أيضا والكسر والجمرة وسائر العلل وليس كذلك حقيقة الأمر لكن على مثال ٦
ما هو جزء من البدن ذلك الذى يقال له آلة قال حنين افهم عنده قوله
آلة فى هذا الموضع آلة على الطريق العامّ كذلك هو جزء من الطبّ
معرفة شفاء الورم على مثال ما العين جزء من البدن على ذلك المثال بعينه معرفة
شفاء الرمد جزء من الطبّ وأعنى بالرمد ورما ما يحدث فى اللباس الخارج عن
سائر لباس العين وهذا المرض إذا كان فى الرئة يسمّى ذات الرئة وإذا كان فى
الغشاء المستبطن للأضلاع سمّى ذات الجنب فإنّ هذه العلل إنّما هى أورام
ما تحدث فى أعضاء ما والحيلة فى شفاء الورم الذى يقال على الطريق الجنسىّ غير
الحيلة فى شفاء الورم المحدود فى أىّ عضو هو كما أنّ الآلة التى تقال على
الطريق الجنسىّ هى غير الآلة التى تقال على طريق التلخيص إذ كانت الحيلة
لمداواة الورم غير الحيلة لمداواة الورم الحادث فى هذا العضو المشار إليه كما بيّنت
فى مقالاتى من كتاب حيلة البرء

٥ وليس يزعم صاحب التجربة أنّ مداواة ما جنسيّة تعقل للورم على انفراده
إلّا أنّه على حال على رأى هذا أيضا ليس على مثال ما يتوهّم توهّم الورم كذلك

17 على[I]] *fort.* وعلى *legendum est* 21 الورم] الورم المحدود Ms.: *corr.* S'

produce inflammation in the layers that he is piercing and communicate the pain in the eye to the whole head. In order to prevent this from happening one needs the preparatory art, whose aim must be to clear the whole body of superfluities and to allay the pains in the head. The sciences that lead to these results are the elements of the art of medicine, as are those that preserve the eyes from inflammation after the cataract has been couched and keep the head free from pain. By this I mean that these are amongst the *ultimate and the minutest* parts of medicine.

This argument that I have used must be applied by analogy to all 5
ailments. The knowledge of the cure of each of them, whichever it may be, will be a part of the art of medicine in the same way that the so-called organs are parts of the animal body. *But here we must deal with a possible source of error before* completing our summary of this whole topic. It may be thought that, as there is an art devoted to the cure of cataracts, there should be another to cure inflammation, treated absolutely – *Ḥunain said: What he says here should be understood as applying to the inflammation produced from the blood, which is known to the Greeks as flegmonē. This is the only type to which they apply the term "inflammation" absolutely.* –, and, in the same way, others should deal with ulcers, fractures, erysipelas and the other ailments. In fact, however, this is not so. Rather, in the same way that the so- 6
called organ – *Ḥunain said: His use of the term organ in this context must be understood as following common usage.* – is part of the body, the knowledge of the cure of inflammation is part of the art of medicine and so, as the eye is part of the body, the knowledge of the cure of ophthalmia, by which I mean inflammation affecting the eye's outer tunic, is part of this art. When this disease affects the lung it is called pneumonia and when it affects the inner costal membrane it is called pleurisy, as these ailments are simply inflammations produced in certain parts. What is used to cure inflammation, when this term is used generically, differs from the cures of specific instances of it that affect certain parts of the body, whichever these may be, just as the generic term "organ" differs from a specified organ. For the methods used to treat inflammation differ from those that are used to treat the inflammation that has affected a definite limb, as I showed in what I wrote in my "On Therapeutic Methods".

5. The Empiricists do not consider that any generic treatment can be understood as applying to inflammation by itself. *However, even*

يتوهّم توهّم الماء فى العين لأنّ العضو فى هذه العلّة التى حدثت فيه الآن محدود
وليس هو محدودا فى الورم وليس تضطرّنا الأمور فى التبيين بأكثر من هذا حتّى
نرقّق فى أشباه هذه من الأشياء الفكر والقول لكنّا نجمل القول فى جملة واحدة ٢
فنقول انّ الطبّ بالجملة هو معرفة شفاء الأمراض وينقسم إلى أقسام أول هى أولى
الأقسام وهى معرفة شفاء الأمراض المفردة والبسيطة وبعدها شفاء الأمراض المركّبة
ثمّ بعدها الأمراض التى فى أجزاء من البدن أمّا أوّلا ففى أجزاء بسيطة مفردة ثمّ
من بعد فى أجزاء مركّبة وقد بيّنت فى مقالة أفردتها فى تصنيف الأمراض فعنونتها
فى أصناف الأمراض كم هى الأمراض البسيطة المفردة وكم هى المركّبة وإذ كان ٣
شأن الطبّ ألّا يقتصر على إزالة الأبدان عن الأمراض إلى الصحّة لكن من شأنه
أيضا أن يحفظ على الأصحّاء صحّتهم كما بيّنت فى مقالة أخرى صار جزءا
آخر من صناعة الطبّ يقال له حفظ الصحّة يوضع فى القسمة بإزاء الجزء الذى
تقدّم ذكره وهو الجزء الشافى ويصير لهذا الجزء أيضا أجزاء أخر وهى أصناف
المعارف التى بها يحفظ كلّ واحد من أعضاء البدن على صحّته وإن كانت أيضا ٤
حال أخرى ثالثة للبدن موجودة وهى التى لا ننسبها لا إلى الصحّة ولا إلى المرض
فقد يجب ضرورة أن يكون هذا أيضا جزءا آخر من هذه الصناعة يشتمل عليها
عنايتها وهذه الحال قد يظنّ أنّها حال مَن بدنه قد اضطرب اضطرابا بيّنا إلّا أنّه
لم يمرض بعد لكنّه يقدر أن يفعل أفعاله على العادة أو ليست به بليّة محسوسة
لكن به بليّة لا تحسّ مثل من قد عضّه الكلب الكلِب أو سقى دواء قتّالا إنّما
شأنه أن يقتل فى حال ما وبعد مدّة من الزمان طويلة فإن لهذه الأحوال قد ٥
يظنّ أنّ لها جزءا خاصّا مرتّبا لمداواتها وهو التقدّم فى حفظ الصحّة وكذلك الأمر
فيمن كان قد خرج عن الحمّى مثلا منذ قريب إلّا أنّه بعد ضعيف يمنعه ضعفه
عن أن يستحمّ وحده من غير معاون فقد أقيم له من صناعة الطبّ جزء يقال له
التلافى والجزء أيضا الذى يسمّى تدبير المشائخ قد يظنّ أنّه مرتّب لحال البدن ٦
الذى ليس بصحيح ولا مريض إذ كانت الشيخوخة ليس هى مرضا بالحقيقة ولا
صحّة كاملة مستحكمة وقد رتّب قوم فى هذا الموضع ذلك الجزء الذى يسمّى ٧

11 *post* الطبّ *fort.* جزء *inserendum est* 15 يكون هذا *sic* 19 لهذه *sic, ut vid.*: *melius* هذه

following this view, the concept of inflammation cannot be thought of as the same as that of a cataract. For in this latter case the part of the body affected by the ailment now is defined, whereas this was not so in the case of inflammation. There is no necessity to clarify this point any further so as to exercise subtlety of thought and speech in matters like this.

To sum up, then, in a single sentence, we say that medicine, seen as 2
a whole, is the knowledge of the cure of diseases. It is split into its primary and most appropriate divisions, which consist of the knowledge of the cure, firstly of the individual and simple diseases, next of the compound diseases and next of those that affect certain parts of the body, firstly simple and then compound parts. I have written a treatise devoted to the classification of disease, called "On the Types of Disease", in which I have shown how many simple and how many compound diseases there are.

Medicine, of course, does not confine itself to bringing bodies from 3
sickness to health but it is also concerned with preserving the healthy in their health, as I showed in another treatise. So it has another division called "the preservation of health," which is on a par with the branch that has already been mentioned, that is the therapeutic. This part also has further sub-divisions that form the branches of knowledge by which the health of individual bodily parts is preserved.
If there is, besides this, a third physical condition related neither to 4
health nor to sickness, this too must form another branch of medicine and be included in medical practice. Such a condition is, in fact, held to be that of a man whose physical balance is plainly upset, though he is not yet ill and can still function normally. It may be that there is nothing perceptible wrong with him although he has some hidden complaint. For example, he may have been bitten by a mad dog or have drunk something deadly whose function it is to kill only in certain
circumstances and after a long period of time. Some think that there 5
is a special division of the art of medicine devoted to the cure of these states, this being the prophylactic. The same type of thing applies, for example, to those who have recently recovered from *fever* and are still so weak that they cannot wash by themselves without help. For these people have devoted to them a branch of the art of medicine
known as the recuperative. The so-called treatment of the elderly is 6
also thought to be designed to deal with the condition of a body that is *neither healthy nor sick*. For old age is not, properly speaking, a disease
nor is it perfect, sound, health. Some people have inserted here that 7

تدبير الصبيان أعنى فى خلال أجزاء الصناعة التى تعنى بالبدن التى شأنها القصد
للعناية بحال الأبدان التى ليست بصحيحة ولا مريضة وهاهنا جزء آخر مع هذه
بحفظ خصب البدن بعضهم يسمّيه خصب البدن وبعضهم يسمّيه فنّ الدلك
حتّى تكون أجزاء الصناعة التى تعنى بالبدن الأول التى هى أعظم أجزائها الجزء ٨
الشافى وجزء التلافى وجزء التقدّم فى الحفظ للصحّة وجزء تدبير المشائخ وجزء
تدبير الصبيان وجزء حفظ الصحّة وجزء حفظ خصب البدن وهذه الأجزاء أيضا
كلّها إذا قسمت كما بيّنّا آنفا من قسمة الجزء الشافى صارت إلى أصناف
العلوم المفردة البسيطة التى لا تنقسم إلى غيرها وهى التى قلنا انّها أركان صناعة
الطبّ

٦ فهذا الطريق بأسره من القسمة يجرى بحسب حالات الأبدان ولصناعة
الطبّ صنف آخر من القسمة يجرى بحسب أصناف الأعمال فى صناعة الطبّ
وذلك متى قالوا انّ أجزاء صناعة الطبّ الأول التى هى فى غاية العظم هى العلاج
باليد واستعمال الأدوية والتدبير وقد يظنّ بعض الناس أنّه قد يمكن أن يجرى هذا
الطريق من القسمة بحسب مادّة الأسباب وذلك أنّ جميع ما من شأنه أن يجلب على
البدن المرض أو يفيده الصحّة إنّما يبتدئ إمّا من التدبير وإمّا من الأدوية وإمّا
من العلاج باليد لكنّ الأولى أن يقال فى ذلك أنّ جميع ما من شأنه أن يفعل
ذلك فى البدن إنّما هو من الأشياء التى تتناول فترد البدن والأشياء التى تفعل بالبدن
والأشياء التى تستفرغ من البدن والأشياء التى تلقاه من خارج فيكون القائل لذلك قد
قسم مادّة الأسباب وأنا أختصر القول فى ذلك فأجمله فأقول انّ قوما جعلوا قسمة ٢
جملة الطبّ إلى أجزائه الملائمة من الحالات التى من شأن صناعة الطبّ إصلاحها
وشفاؤها وحفظها فحكموا بأنّ عدد أجزاء هذه الصناعة كعدد أصناف حالات
البدن وقوما لم يقتصروا على أن جعلوا قسمة الطبّ إلى أجزائه من هذه فقط لكن
من المادّة بأسرها التى عند الطبيب معرفتها فأضافوا إلى الأجزاء التى ذكرناها جزء
الكلام الطبيعىّ وجزء الكلام فى الاسباب والجزء الذى يخصّ بأن يسمّى الموادّىّ
فعدّوها معها وقوما قسموا أجزاء الطبّ من أفعالها كلّها واضافوا إلى التدبير
واستعمال الأدوية والعلاج باليد استخراج الدلائل أيضا وقوما قسموا استخراج

3^II خصب البدن] *melius* حفظ خصب البدن   14 على] عن *emendaverit* Strohmaier   21 حالات] الات Ms.

branch known as paediatrics – I mean, they have included it amongst those branches of medical care of the body that have as their object the treatment of the condition of those who are neither healthy nor sick. Besides these there is yet another part that concerns itself with the preservation of eutrophy and which is known to some as eutrophy and to others as the art of *massage*.

The prime and main branches, then, of the art that concerns itself 8
with the body are these: the therapeutic, the recuperative, the prophylactic, the geriatric, the paediatric, together with those that are concerned with the preservation *of health and of eutrophy*. These branches may all be subdivided, as we showed earlier in our division of the therapeutic, and this leads to the types of the simple and indivisible sciences of which we have said that they are the elements of medicine.

6. This whole method of division follows the differences in physical states. But medicine has another type of division that is based on the various classes of operation performed in it, as when one says that its primary and main branches are those of surgery, pharmacy and diet. It has been thought by some that this kind of division can be based on *material causes*, in that everything whose function it is *to bring illness to the body* or to give it health has its origin either in diet, drugs or surgery. Yet it is better to say on that point that whatever affects the body like this must be one of the things that are taken by it, that act upon it, that are evacuated from it, or that meet it externally. For whoever says that has produced a division of material causes.

I shall abbreviate and summarise the argument here and say that 2
some people have divided all medicine into the parts that correspond to the conditions that it has to rectify, to cure, or to preserve. They have then given it as their judgement that there are as many branches to the art of medicine as there are bodily states. Others have not confined themselves to this division but have added branches taken from the whole range of what comes within the doctor's cognisance. So over and above those that we have mentioned they have included physiology together with *aetiology and* what is particularised as the material section, all of which they have counted in with the others. Then there are those whose division is based on all the operations of medicine. To regimen, *pharmacy and surgery* they have added diagnosis, which others, in turn, have subdivided into what deals with the forms of

الدلائل إلى صور العلل وإلى تقدمة المعرفة فأضافوا هذين إلى الأجزاء الثلاثة التى
تقدّم ذكرها وأمّا أكثر أصحاب التجربة كما قلت فإنّهم لمّا أن قالوا انّ ٣
الأجزاء المتمّمة هى استخراج الدلائل والشفاء والجزء الذى يسمّى حفظ الصحّة
جعلوا أجزاء الشفاء فى قسمتهم له التدبير والعلاج باليد واستعمال الأدوية
فأخطؤوا فى التسمية وذلك أنّه قد كان يجب عليهم أن يذكروا فى هذا الموضع
أسماء العلوم لا أسماء الأفعال ولم يخطؤوا فى الأمور أنفسها فالأولى أن يقال ٤
كما قد يقول القليل منهم انّ لصناعة الطبّ جزءا يستخرج الدلائل ولها جزء
آخر هو الشافى وجزءها الآخر هو الحافظ للصحّة وانّ جزء المستخرج للدليل منه
تصوير العلل ومنه تقدمة الإنذار وعلى هذا المثال فإنّ الجزء الشافى منه جزء مدبّر
ومنه جزء يستعمل الأدوية ومنه جزء يستعمل العلاج باليد ولك أن تسمّى هذه
الأجزاء التى ذكرناها كلّها علوما أيضا فتقول انّ هاهنا علما شافيا وعلما
مستعملا للعلاج باليد وعلما مدبّرا وسائر أجزاء جملة الطبّ النظائر لهذه
الأجزاء وإن قلت مكان العلم معرفة أو حكمة أو باب نظر فلا عليك إذ كان
ليس بين ذلك اختلاف فإنّة ليس قصدك تتبّع الأسماء لكنّ الوقوف على معرفة
أصناف الأمور وأمّا اعتقادهم أنّ أجزاء الطبّ بالجملة الأول الجنسيّة صنفان ٥
فقد أصابوا فى قولهم ذلك غاية الصواب وذلك أنّ أجزاء الطبّ بعضها متمّمة
وبعضها مقوّمة فالأجزاء المتمّمة هى الأجزاء التى بها يكون قوام غاية الطبّ
والأجزاء المقوّمة لهذه الأجزاء هى أجزاء أخر وهى أسباب قوامها وكأنّها
أصناف وجودها وأمّا ترتيبهم استخراج الدلائل مع الجزء الشافى والجزء الحافظ ٦
للصحّة حتّى سوّوا بينه وبينهما فى القدر والمرتبة فلم يصيبوا فى ذلك فإنّ
استخراج الدلائل متقدّم ضرورة للشفاء وحفظ الصحّة من قبل أنّه ليس
يمكن أحد أن يحفظ صحّة إنسان من الناس ولا أن يشفيه من غير أن يعرف
حال بدنه كيف هى لكن ليس إنّما تمّ الغاية المقصود إليها بالطبّ عن
استخراج الدلائل نفسه ومع ذلك فإنّ الانتقال من الشىء إلى نظيره ليس هو أيضا
جزءا مساويا فى القدر والمرتبة للعيان والخبر لكن ليس يحتاج فى هذا القول منّى إلى
بيان فى هذا الموضع وذلك أنّ قسيس النظار قد بلغ فى تبيين ذلك فى مقالة بأسرها
ولم يكن سارافس من أصحاب التجربة يخالف فى هذا المعنى فمن كان قصده

8 جزء المستخرج *sic* 26 قسيس] قسبس Ms.

disease as well as into prognosis. These two divisions they have then
added to the three mentioned above.

As for the Empiricists, most of them, *as I said*, have taken the per- 3
fective parts to be the diagnostic, the therapeutic and what is known
as the preservation of health. The subdivisions of the therapeutic
section they have marked off as diet, *surgery and pharmacy*. However,
they have made a mistake in their terminology, for what they should
have done here was to mention the names of the sciences and not of
the actions. They were not mistaken, however, in the points themselves.
It would, then, be best to say, as a few of them do, that the art of 4
medicine has a diagnostic branch together with one that is therapeutic
and a final one that deals with the preservation of health. Of the
diagnostic branch, one section deals with the distinction of ailments
and another with prognosis. Similarly the therapeutic branch has one
section that deals with *diet*, another with pharmacy and a third with
surgery. *All these parts that we have mentioned you can, if you want,
call sciences and you can say that there is here one science relating to
cures, another relating to surgery and a third to diet, and the same thing
applies to other similar parts of the whole art of medicine. You are not
wrong, though, if you talk of "knowledge" or "wisdom" or "theory" in
place of "science", as there is no difference between these terms. Nor are
you concerned to follow up names but to reach an understanding of the
categories involved.*

As for the belief of the Empiricists that the primary and generic 5
branches of medicine, treated as a whole, are of two types, in this they
are entirely right. For the parts of medicine are either perfective or
constitutive. It is through the former that medicine achieves its ob-
jects, while the constitutive parts of these are different and are, in
fact, the causes of their constitution and, as it were, the classes of their
existence. They are not right, however, in putting the diagnostic branch on 6
a par in importance with the therapeutic and with that which deals with
the preservation of health. For diagnosis must necessarily precede the
other two, as it is not possible to preserve anyone's health or to cure
him without knowing the state of his body. However, the object aimed
at in medicine is not to be achieved just by simple diagnosis. Nor is
differential diagnosis a section equal in importance to inspection and
information. There is no need for me to give any explanation of this
point here as it was shown clearly *by Cassius the theoretician* in a
whole treatise devoted to this subject and the point was not opposed

أن يعرف ذلك ممّن يسلك سبيل التجربة فلينظر فى تلك المقالة وأمّا أنا فلأنّى
أعلم من مذهبك أنّك تقصد السبيل التى تؤدّى إلى الشفاء بطريق الاستدلال
والقياس فأنا جاعل ابتداء ذلك شبيها بما يبتدئ به أصحاب التجربة ثمّ أقبل على
ما يتّصل بذلك

٧ فأقول انّ أجزاء الطبّ بعضها خاصّيّة أول أولى الأجزاء بها وهذه الأجزاء
هى التى بها تمّ الغاية المقصود إليها من هذه الصناعة وبعضها تتقدّم هذه
ضرورة وبعضها يتقدّم أيضا مرتبتها تلك الأجزاء المتقدّمة فالأجزاء الخاصّيّة الأول
التى هى أولى الأجزاء فعددها كعدد أصناف مادّة الطبّ وأولى الموادّ بالطبّ
حالات أبداننا كانت اثنتين أوثلث أو أكثر من ذلك وقد بيّنت فى المقالة التى ٢
وسمتها باسم ثراسوبلس أنّ الأصناف الأول من حالات الأبدان صنفان لهما
اسمان يخصّانهما عند جميع الناس فمن عادتنا أن نسمّى أحدهما الصحّة
ونسمّى الآخر المرض ولكلّ واحد من هذين الصنفين أيضا نوعان وذلك أنّ
كلّ واحد من الصحّة والمرض إمّا أن يكون موجودا على طريق الثبات والتمكّن
وإمّا أن يكون موجودا على طريق الإضافة والأجزاء التى تعنى بالصحّة الموجودة ٣
على طريق الثبات والتمكّن تسمّى الحافظ للصحّة وهذا هو الجزء الذى جعل
بعض الناس حفظ خصب البدن جزءا خاصّيّا له والأجزاء من صناعة الطبّ التى
تعنى بالصحّة الموجودة على طريق الإضافة هى الجزء الذى يتقدّم فى حفظ الصحّة
وجزء تلافى الصحّة وجزء تدبير المشائخ وأمّا أجزاء صناعة الطبّ التى تقصد بعناية
المرض الموجود على طريق الثبات والتمكّن والمرض الموجود على طريق الإضافة
فليست لها أسماء على أنّ بعض الأمراض قد تسمّى مزمنة وبعضها حادّة
فهذه هى أجزاء هذه الصناعة الأول وأولى الأجزاء بها فأمّا الأجزاء التى لا ٤
يمكن وجود هذه دونها فأولها المستخرجة للدلائل ولهذه جزآن أحدهما المتعرّف
للأشياء الحاضرة والآخر المنذر بالأشياء الكائنة وذلك أنّه ليس يمكن أحد من غير
أن يكون قد عرف المرض أن يقف على علاجه ولا يمكنه أن يعالجه على ما ينبغى من
غير أن يكون قد عرف مدّة إتيان البحران وصورة المرض وقد يتقدّم هذين
الجزأين ضرورة أجزاء أخر أحدها العلم بالأعضاء كلّها وذلك يدرك بتشريح
الموتى والثانى العلم بأفعالها والثالث العلم بمنافعها وهذان أيضا يدركان بالعلم

5 أولى] اول Ms., ut vid. 8 أولى الأجزاء] اجزاء Ms.: اول الاجزاء S¹
10 وسمتها sic: sed cf. p. 48,6 رسمتها 15 الحافظ sic

by Serapio *the Empiricist. Those Empiricists* who wish to learn this
should study that treatise. As for me, I know that the course that you
follow is to try to find a path leading to a knowledge of therapy by
deduction and *analogy*. I shall, then, take as my starting point one
which resembles that of the Empiricists and go on from there to what
follows next.

7. I say that of the parts of the art of medicine some are *peculiar,*
primary and proper and these are the parts through which this art
achieves its object. *Other parts necessarily precede these* and there are
others that precede the preceding ones in position. As for the first
group, the number of its parts is that of the divisions of the subjects
of medicine, whose matter may most properly be taken to be physical
states, whether there be two, three or more of these. In the treatise 2
that I named after Thrasyboulos I showed that there are two
primary types of the states of the human body, which are particularised
by two names that are in general use. For habitually we call one of
them health and the other disease. Each one of these two classes has
two subdivisions, as both health and disease can be either firmly rooted
or else found as something superimposed. The sections of medicine 3
that deal with health in the first of these categories are called those
that preserve health and it is as a special subdivision of this that some
have posited the preservation of eutrophy. *As for what deals with*
health in the second category, this comprises prophylaxis, the recuperative
branch and that of geriatrics. When it comes to disease in the first and
second categories, the parts of medicine whose object is to deal with
this have no names, though some diseases are called chronic and others
acute.

These are the primary parts into which medicine may most properly 4
be divided. There are others, however, without which these branches
cannot exist, the first being the diagnostic. This has two sub-divisions,
the first being the recognition of what is present and the second prognosis of what is to come. For nobody can find out how to treat a
disease until he knows what it is. Nor can he treat it properly
until he knows when its crisis will come *or what shape the*
disease will take. These two sections are, in turn, necessarily preceded
by others. One of these is the knowledge of all the parts of the body,
which is something that is learnt by dissecting dead bodies. One must,
however, know, secondly, the actions of the bodily parts and, thirdly,
their uses, these being things that can be understood through a know-

بأمر اسطقسات البدن ثمّ بعلم أمر أصناف المزاج ثمّ بالعلم ثالثا بأمر القوى الطبيعيّة والقوى النفسانيّة مع تشريح الأحياء فإنّ استخراج الدلائل إلى هذه المبادئ يمكن أن يحلّ وهى التى قلت انّها متقدّمة لا محالة للشفاء ولحفظ الصحّة فقد بيّنت ذلك كلّه فى الكتب التى خصّصتها لها وهاهنا جزء آخر للطبّ ٥
قرين للجزء المستخرج للدليل يتقدّم الجزء الشافى وهو المعرفة بأسباب الصحّة والمرض كلّها وهذا العلم هو الذى يسمّيه بعض الناس الموادّىّ وبه تعرف موادّ الأسباب كلّها وموادّ الأسباب مصوّرة فى الأشياء التى ترد البدن والأشياء التى تفعل به والأشياء التى تستفرغ منه والأشياء التى تلقاه من خارج حتّى تنظر فى قوّة كلّ واحد من هذه الأشياء التى ذكرناها فتعرفها وقد بيّنت فى كتابى فى حيلة البرء ما الحاجة إلى هذه فى صناعة الطبّ

٨ فهذا هو الطريق إلى إدراك صناعة الطبّ بحسب المادّة التى هى أولى الموادّ بها وأمّا السبيل إلى إدراك أجزائها التى هى بحسب المادّة التى هى أولى بها على الطريق الثانى فتجرى على هذا النحو أقول انّ بدن الإنسان هو مادّة ثانية لصناعة الطبّ وكأنّه مادّة لها على طريق العرض وذلك أنّ الصحّة والمرض إنّما هما حالات البدن فإنّ بدن الإنسان هو مادّة ثانية ومادّة على طريق العرض للفلسفة الطبيعيّة ٢
أيضا إذ كان قابلا للكون والفساد وكانت الفلسفة الطبيعيّة إنّما شأنها البحث عن ما هو قابل للكون والفساد ولذلك صارت المادّة الأولى لهذه أيضا الكون ومن قبل ذلك صار مادّتها على طريق العرض الجسم المتكوّن أيضا فإنّ بدن الإنسان أيضا إنّما صار مادّة للعلم الطبيعىّ من طريق أنّه قابل للكون والفساد وليس من هذه الطريق صار مادّة لصناعة الطبّ لكن من طريق أنّه قابل للآلام والفساد فلمّا ٣
كان بدن الإنسان كأنّه مادّة لصناعة الطبّ فإنّ صناعة الطبّ تنقسم من الأجزاء على قدر ما يحتمل البدن من القسمة فتكون أصنافها الأول الجنسيّة صنفين أحدهما فى الأعضاء التى تجرى مجرى الأركان والأخرى ‹ فى › الأعضاء الآليّة وإذا قسمنا هذه بأجزائها كانت أجزاء الطبّ على قدر عدد أعضاء البدن التى تجرى مجرى الأركان والأعضاء الآليّة وعلى قدر علل كلّ واحد منها وذلك أنّ كلّ واحد من علل كلّ واحد من الأعضاء يصير له من الطبّ جزء يخصّه

7 مصوّرة *sic, ut vid.* : *vel* متصوّرة *legendum est?* 20 والفساد *sic* : *fort. sec. Lat.* والشفاء *corrigendum est* 23 فى *supplevi*

ledge of the elements of the body and the varieties of its *compounding*, as well as through a third science, that of the natural *and spiritual* forces, which is accompanied by the dissection of living things. For the diagnostic branch of medicine can be resolved into these principals and it is of these that I have said that they have to precede therapy and the preservation of health. With all these points I have dealt clearly in the books that I have devoted to them.

But there is here another branch of medicine that is on a par with 5
the diagnostic and precedes the therapeutic. This is the knowledge of all the causes of health and sickness and it is this that some people call the material part of medicine. Through it can be learnt all the *material* causes, *which* take their form in what comes into the body, what acts on it, what is evacuated from it and what meets it externally. The powers of each one of these things that I have mentioned are to be studied and recognised, and I have clearly explained in my work "On Therapeutic Methods" what the medical need for them is.

8. This, then, is the way to grasp the art of medicine in accordance
with its own special material. But the way to grasp the branches
into which it is divided and which are secondary in relation to this
material is as follows. I say that the human body provides secondary 2
and, as it were, accidental material for the art of medicine. For health
and disease are simply bodily states. The body also serves, in a secondary
and accidental way, as material for natural philosophy in that it is
capable of generation and corruption and the sole business of natural
philosophy is to investigate this class of things. Thus its primary
matter is generation and for that reason material is supplied it *acci-
dentally* by the generated body. So the reason why the human body
becomes the matter for natural science is because it is subject to
generation and corruption, but this is not the way in which it becomes
matter for the art of medicine. Rather, it does so because of its liability
to pain and to *corruption*.

Therefore, as the human body is, as it were, material for the art of 3
medicine, this art can be split into as many parts as those into which the body can be divided. It will have two *prime* generic types, one being found in the elementary parts and the other in those that are organic. *When we divide these with all their subdivisions, the number of the sections of medicine will be that of these two classes of parts with the ailments that can affect each of them added in.* For each one of these ailments of each one of these parts has a division of medicine peculiar

وقـد بيّنّـا أنّ جزءا جزءا من هذه الأجزاء ينقسم إلى العلاجـات الجزئيّة فى
ذكرنا لأمر قدح الماء فإنّ العلم بهذه هو أجزاء هذه الصناعة بأسرها التى تجرى
مجرى الأركان وأمّا فى العلل التى يكون شفاؤها بالأدوية فالعلم بكلّ واحد من
الأدوية المفردة وكذلك أيضا فى العلل التى يكون برؤها بالتدبير العلم بأصناف
التدبير البسيطة وليس من هذه المادّة وحدهـا قـد تنحطّ القسمة إلى الأجزاء ٤
الأواخر التى تجرى مجرى الاسطقسات من هذه الصناعة لكن قد ينحطّ أيضا إليها
من القسمة التى ذكرناهـا قبيل وكذلك أيضا إذا أجريت القسمة على وجه آخر أىّ
وجه كان فلننزل أنّا قصدنا لأن نقسم جنسا من أجناس الحالات إلى التى تنتهى ٥
إلى أجزائها الأواخر ونجعل ذلك الجنس جنس المرض فتكون القسمة الأولى فى هذا
الجنس أن نقول انّ بعض الأمراض تعرض فى الأعضاء المتشابهة الأجزاء وبعضها
فى الأعضاء الآليّة على ما بيّنّا فى المقالة التى وضعناها فى أصناف الأمراض
والقسمة الثانية أنّ بعض الأمراض بسيطة وبعضها مركّبة على ما بيّنّا أيضا
من ذلك فى تلك المقالـة فالعلم بشفـاء واحد من هذه الأمراض أيّها كان قد ٦
يحتاج فيه إلى العلم بالأجزاء التى ليس وراءها غاية فى الصغر الجارية مجرى
الاسطقسات وهى تلك الأجزاء التى تقدّم ذكرها فلننزل مثلا أنّا قصدنا لشفاء
مرض حارّ فلا نعلم أنّا لا محالة نحتاج أوّلا فى شفائه أن نعلم أنّ الأضداد هى
شفاء لأضدادها فإنّ ذلك قد تبيّن أنّه هو العلم الشامل العامّ المتقدّم لجميع
العلوم بأصناف الشفاء ثمّ من بعد ذلك نحتاج أن نعلم أنّ المرض الحارّ إنّما
ينبغى أن يشفى بالأشياء المبرّدة ثمّ من بعد ذلك أنّ المرض الحارّ فى الدرجة
الأولى مثلا إنّما ينبغى أن يشفى بما هو بارد فى الدرجة الأولى ثمّ من بعد ذلك نحتاج
أن نعلم مراتب الأمراض الحارّة فى الدرج ومراتب الأدوية المبرّدة على ما بيّنّا
فى كتبنا فى الأدوية فقد يعلّم ذلك أنّ الإنسان من حيث ابتدأ بالقسمة فإنّه إذا ٧
سلك فيها سبيل الصواب إلى أن ينتهى إلى العلوم الأواخر التى تجرى مجرى الأركان
فإنّ القسمة تؤدّيه إلى العلوم التى تقدّم ذكرها
٩ وكيما تقف على هذا المعنى فيضح لك بأكثر ممّا وضح فأنا ذاكر شيئا
من الأقسام الأخر وخاصّة القسمة التى استعملناها مرارا كثيرة فأقول انّ الأشياء
الموجودة فى بدن الحيوان بعضها طبيعيّة وبعضها خارجة عن الطبيعة والأشياء
الخارجة عن الطبيعة بعضها هى أمراض وبعضها أعراض لازمة للأمراض وبعضها

8 التى تنتهى] أن ننتهى *emendaverit* Strohmaier 21 المبرّدة] المفردة Ms.

to it. We have shown how each of these separate divisions can be subdivided into treatments of individual parts in our account of cataracts, and a knowledge of these things represents all the elementary divisions of this art. As for the ailments that can be cured by the use of drugs, here the relevant science is that of all the simples, and where the ailments are to be cured by diet, it is that of the simple forms of diet.

However, it is not this material side alone that brings our division 4
to the final and elementary parts of medicine, as this is also achieved by the division that we mentioned earlier and the same thing happens if any other method of division is used. Let us suppose that we are 5
intending to split one of the classes of physical conditions so as to arrive at its ultimate sections and let us suppose that this condition is that of disease. The first thing to do in subdividing it is to say that some diseases occur in the homoiomerous parts and others in those that are organic, as we showed in our treatise "On the Types of Disease". Secondly we can say that some diseases are simple and others compound, as we also showed there. So the knowledge of how 6
to cure any one of these diseases requires a knowledge of the minutest, the elementary, parts, which are those that we have already mentioned. Let us suppose, for instance, that we want to cure a hot disease without realising that first, to cure it, we need to know that opposites cure opposites. For it has been clearly shown that this knowledge is the all-embracing general preliminary to everything that is known about types of therapy. Secondly, we have to know that a hot disease must be treated by what is cooling and next that a first degree hot disease, for example, must be treated by what is cooling to a similar degree. After that you must know the various subsequent stages of hot diseases and of cooling drugs, as I have shown in my books on drugs.

The lesson of this is that, wherever you start your division, if you 7
follow it properly until you reach the ultimate and elemental sciences, you will find that it will bring you to those that we have already mentioned.

9. In order that you should understand this and have it clarified even further, I shall mention some of the other divisions and especially the one that I have often used. I say that of what is to be found in the animal body some things are natural and some unnatural. Of the latter some are diseases, some the symptoms that accompany disease and

أسباب الأمراض فأمّا الأشياء الطبيعيّة فينبغى أن يكون عند الطبيب العلمُ
بحفظها وأمّا الأشياء الخارجة عن الطبيعة فينبغى أن يكون عنده العلم بإزالتها
وصرفها وليس هذا موضع ذكر السبل التى يوصل بها إلى كلّ واحد من هذين
الأمرين إذ كنّا قد بيّنّا ذلك فى مواضع أخر وغرضى فى هذا الموضع أن أعدّد ٢
كلّ واحد من الأشياء التى ذكرتها فأقسمه القسمة التى هى أولى به إلّا أنّى قد
كتبت فى كلّ واحد منها فكتبت فى الأمراض فى المقالة التى رسمتها فى أصناف
الأمراض وكتبت فى الأسباب أيضا على انفرادها مقالة أخرى وكذلك أيضا فإنّى
كتبت فى الأعراض مقالة أخرى وذكرت أصناف الأبدان الصحيحة كلّها فى ٣
كتابى فى حفظ الأصحّاء وذكرت فيه أيضا كيف ينبغى أن يعنى بكلّ واحد
منها وحللناها إلى أن بلغنا إلى العلوم المفردة التى تجرى مجرى الأركان وكذلك أيضا
فعلنا فى أمر الأمراض والأسباب والأعراض فى كتابنا فى حيلة البرء فإنّ فى هذه ٤
القسمة أيضا الأجزاء الأول لهذه الصناعة والتى هى أولى الأجزاء بها ليس توجد
غير تلك التى ذكرناها آنفا وكذلك أيضا الأجزاء التى هى أول على الطريق الثانى
والتى هى أول على الطريق الثالث على ما ذكرنا وانّ هذه أيضا قد ينبغى أن تقسم
إلى أن نبلغ بها إلى البسيطة المفردة التى ليس وراءها غاية فإنّ الإنسان من حيث
ابتدأ بالقسمة إذا سلك فيها سبيل الصواب فقسمته تؤدّى لا محالة إلى العلوم
التى تجرى مجرى الأركان وأمّا أن للإنسان أن يقسم كلّ واحد من الأمور التى ٥
توضع للقسمة على وجوه كثيرة فلم يقتصر الحذّاق من الفلاسفة ومن يتقدّم
سائرهم فى البلاغة على أن قالوا ذلك قولا مجرّدا لكن قد مثّله قوم منهم كما
فعل فلاطن فى مقالتين بأسرهما إحداهما موسومة بسوفسطيس والأخرى
فوليطيقوس فليس ينبغى لك أن ترتاب لكثرة التقسيم ولا تجعل نظرك وتفقّدك ٦
من أمر من تقدّمنا هل قسموا الطبّ بطرق مختلفة بل هل أتوا على جميع ما
يحتوى عليه فلم يبقوا شيئا فإنّ من لزم ذلك كان قد سلك فى القسمة سبيل
القصد والأفضل على ما قلت آنفا أن تجعل مبدأ القسمة من المادّة التى هى
أولى الموادّ ثمّ عند ذلك تضيف إليها سائر أصناف القسمة على الطريق والسبيل
التى ذكرناها

20 موسومة] *an* مرسومة Ms. ? 26 *in fine add.* تمت مقالة جالينوس فى اجزاء الطب وذلك فى العشر الاول من جمادى الاولى سنة ست وخمسين واربعمائة والحمد لله حق حمده وصلى الله على سيدنا محمد النبى واله وسلم تسليما Ms.

some the causes of disease. As for what is natural, the doctor must have the knowledge of how to preserve this, while he must know how to remove and dispense with what is unnatural. *But this is not the place to mention* how one arrives at these two objects, as we have already dealt clearly with that elsewhere.

Here my object is to enumerate each of the things that I have 2
mentioned and to divide them in the way that most properly applies
to them. But I have already written about each of them. I dealt with
diseases in the treatise that I wrote "On the Types of Disease." I de-
voted another tract to causes separately and in the same way I wrote
yet another on symptoms. As for the sum total of the types of healthy 3
bodies, this I mentioned in my book "On the Preservation of the
Healthy", where I also mentioned how one should treat each of them
and I analysed the problem until I arrived at the simple and elementary
sciences. I did the same with diseases, causes and symptoms in my "On
Therapeutic Methods." For in this division also, the primary parts 4
of the art of medicine and those that have the greatest relevance to it
are found to be none other than the ones that I mentioned at the be-
ginning. The same is true of the main parts in the second and third
classifications, as I have said. For these must be sub-divided as well,
until one reaches what is simple and ultimate. If, then, you begin on a
division and follow it up properly you are bound to reach the ele-
mentary sciences.

As for the theory that what is propounded for division can be 5
divided in a number of ways, the skilled philosophers and those of
them who excel in rhetoric have not confined themselves to stating
that simply, but some of them have given illustrations of it. This, for
instance, is what Plato has done in two whole tracts, one called
"Sophistes" and the other "Politikos". So your doubts should not be 6
aroused by the number of methods of division nor should you investi-
gate the ancients to see whether they differed in their partitions of
medicine but to see whether they brought out all that the subject
comprises without any omissions. For whoever holds to that has
followed the mean in this. The best course is, as I said at the start,
that in your division you should begin from whatever may be the most
proper material and then you should add in all the other classes of
division there may be, using the method that I have mentioned.

CONSPECTVS SIGLORVM

Ms. = Aya Sofya 3725
S' = correctiones primae manus

كتاب جالينوس فى الأسباب الماسكة

GALEN'S BOOK ON COHESIVE CAUSES

كتاب جالينوس في الأسباب الماسكة

١ إنّ أوّل من علمته قال سببا ماسكا من الفلاسفة أصحاب المظلّة وذلك
أنّهم يرون أنّه يتكوّن من الاسطقسات الأربعة الأجسام التي يلقّبها ارسطوطاليس
بالمتشابهة الأجزاء ويصفها فلاطن بالمتكوّنة بدءا وأنّ سائر الأجسام إنّما تركّب
من هذه والاسطقسات أنفسها بعضها يسمّونها هيولانيّة وبعضها يسمّونها فعّالة ٢
وذوات قوى ويقولون انّ الاسطقسات الهيولانيّة متماسكة بالاسطقسات ذوات
القوى فالنار والهواء عندهم ذوا قوّة فعّالان والأرض والماء هيولانيّان ويقولون انّه
إذا وقع الامتزاج فإنّ ذوى القوى ينفذان بأسرهما فى الهيولانيّين بأسرهما أى أنّ
الهواء والنار ينفذان فى الماء والأرض وانّ الهواء بارد والنار حارّة وان من شأن الجوهر
أن يجتمع ويتكاثف عن طبيعة الهواء وأن ينبسط وينحلّ ويأخذ موضعا أوسع عن
طبيعة النار وانّ الاسطقسين الفعّالين لطيفا الأجزاء والاسطقسين الآخرين غليظا
الأجزاء ويسمّون كلّ جوهر لطيف الأجزاء روحا ويزعمون أنّ فعله أن يتماسك به ٣
الأجسام الطبيعيّة وأبدان الحيوان وأعنى بقولى الأجسام الطبيعيّة ما كان تكوّنه عن
الطبيعة لا عن مهنة من مهن الناس مثل النحاس والحجارة والذهب والخشب ومن
أعضاء بدن الحيوان الأعضاء التى يقال لها الأول المتشابهة الأجزاء أعنى العصبة
والعرق الضارب وغير الضارب والغضروف والعظم وسائر ما يجرى هذا المجرى وكما ٤
أنّ الناس يصلون الخشب بعضه ببعض بالغراء والضبّات والمسامير والطين والجبسين
والكلس كذلك نجد الطبيعة توصّل أعضاء البدن كلّها حتّى تتّحد بالغضاريف
والرباطات والأوتار ولك أن تسمّى إن آثرت الأعضاء التى تفعل هذا الاتّصال فى ٥
الأعضاء البسيطة أسبابا ماسكة للأعضاء المركّبة وكذلك لك أن تسمّى بمثل ذلك
الطين والجبسين والكلس وسائر ما يقوم مقامها فى الأجرام التى من خارج التى

1 *ante titulum add. (sic)* بسم الله الرحمن الرحيم استعنت بالله تعلى Ms. *post titulum add.* ترجمة حنين بن اسحاق Ms. 2 من[II] *add.* S' 3 يلقّبها S' : يصفها Ms.

GALEN'S BOOK ON COHESIVE CAUSES

1. The first philosophers of my acquaintance to speak of a cohesive
cause were the Stoics. Their view is that from the four elements are
produced those bodies that Aristotle calls homoiomerous and that
are described by Plato as "the first to be generated", while all other
bodies are simply compounds of these. Of the elements themselves, 2
some they call material and some active and dynamic. They maintain
that the material elements are held together by those that are dynamic,
fire and water being *dynamic and*[1] active in their view, while earth and
water are material. They say that, when the elements are intermingled
the dynamic wholly penetrate the material, that is to say, air and fire
penetrate water and earth. Air is cold and fire is hot. The natural
effect of air is to consolidate and thicken a substance, whereas fire
naturally causes expansion, loosening and widening. The two active
elements have fine parts and the other two thick parts. Every sub- 3
stance with fine parts the Stoics call spirit and they think that the
function of this spirit is to produce cohesion in natural and in animal
bodies. By natural bodies I mean those that are produced by nature
and not by human skill, like copper, *stones*, gold, wood and those parts
of the animal body that are called the primary and homoiomerous
parts, that is, nerves, arteries, veins, cartilages, bones and everything
else of the same sort. Men join bits of wood together with glue, nails, 4
pegs, clay, gypsum and lime. Similarly nature is found connecting all
the parts of the body so as to form a united whole by means of *carti-
lages, ligaments and tendons*. If you like, you can call the parts of the 5
body that produce this *union* in the simple members cohesive causes
of the compounds and the same term can be applied to clay, gypsum,
lime and the other things that serve the same purpose in externals

---

[1] Italics in the text of Galen indicate that the passage is found in a different form in the Latin version.

يوصّلها الناس بالمهنة لا الطبيعة إلّا أنّ أصحاب المظلّة ليس هذه هي التي
يسمّونها الأسباب الماسكة بل الجوهر اللطيف الأجزاء من الجوهر الهيولانيّ

٢ فأمّا اثيناوس الذي من أهل اطاليا فإذ كان أوّل من أنشأ في الطبّ الفرقة
التي تعرف بفرقة أصحاب الروح فقد يشبه مذهبه أن يقول في المرض سببا ماسكا
إذ كان إنّما يبني على فرقة أصحاب المظلّة وذلك أنّه كان تلميذ بوسيدونيس وعنه
أخذ وأمّا سائر الأطبّاء الذين يعتقدون آراء أخر فليس يليق بمذهبهم [أيضا] أن
يطلبوا سببا ماسكا في كلّ واحد من الأمراض ولا يليق بمذهبهم أيضا أن يطلبوا
سببا ماسكا في الأجسام المتشابهة الأجزاء التي هي على حالها الطبيعيّة ولا يجوز
لهم أن يقولوا كما كان اثيناوس يقول انّ أصناف الأسباب الأول التي لا أسباب
أعلى منها في الجنس ثلثة والأصناف الثلثة التي كان يقول بها اثيناوس هي هذه ٢
الأوّل منها صنف الأسباب الماسكة والثاني صنف الأسباب السابقة والثالث تستغرقه
مادّة الأسباب البادئة ويسمّي بالأسباب البادئة ما كان خارجا من البدن ومن شأنه ٣
أن يغيّره تغيرا ما أيّ تغير كان ويسمّي ما ولدته هذه الأسباب في أبداننا ممّا
هو من جنس ما يحدث مرضا ما دام لم يحدث بعد مرضا الأسباب السابقة ويقول
انّ الاستحالات التي تحدث عن هذه الأسباب وعن الأسباب التي من خارج في
الروح الغريزيّ حتّى يرطب أو يجفّ أو يسخن أو يبرد هي أسباب ماسكة للأمراض
وذلك أنّ الروح عنده لنفوذه في الأعضاء المتشابهة الأجزاء يحيلها باستحالته
ويشبّهها بنفسه قال فربّما كان حدوث الأسباب الماسكة عن الأسباب البادئة ٤
دفعة من غير متوسّط وربّما كان حدوثها بتوسّط الأسباب السابقة قال فإنّ
الانسان متى أصابه حرّ الشمس تغيّر الروح الغريزيّ فيه وصار أسخن ممّا كان
ومتى أصابه البرد استحال إلى البرد ومتى كانت هذه الاستحالات يسيرة لم يكن
المرض حلّ بالبدن بعد فمتى بلغ من خروج العضو عن مزاجه الطبيعيّ أن
يضرّ ذلك بفعله فقد حلّ به حينئذ مرض من قبل سوء مزاج وسببه الماسك هو
الروح إمّا لأنّه سخن بأكثر من المقدار وإمّا لأنّه برد وإمّا لأنّه يبس وإمّا
لأنّه رطب وأصحاب هذه الفرقة يسمّون بالأسباب السابقة الأخلاط المتولّدة في ٥
أبداننا متى سخنت أو بردت أو رطبت أو يبست بأكثر من المقدار وذلك أنّهم يرون
أنّ الأعضاء الأصليّة تقبل الاستحالة منها على طول الزمان حتّى تصير على مثل حالها

20 فيه *add.* S¹

which are connected by the skill of man and not by nature. It is not these, however, but rather material substance with fine parts that the Stoics call a cohesive cause.

2. As for Athenaeus the Attalean, he founded the medical school known as that of the Animists. It suits his doctrine to speak of a cohesive cause in illness since he bases himself upon the Stoics and he was a pupil and disciple of Posidonius. But it does not suit the theories of those other doctors who hold different views to look for a cohesive cause in every illness nor to try to find it in the homoiomeries in their natural state and they cannot say, as Athenaeus did, that there are three types of primary cause that are ultimate in their class. Athenaeus' three types are as follows: first that of the cohesive 2
causes, then that of the prior causes while the third type is comprised of the matter of the immediate causes. This latter term is applied to 3
externals *whose function it is to produce some change in the body, whatever this change may be.* If what is thus produced in the body belongs to the class of what causes disease, then, while it has not yet actually given rise to a disease, it is known as a prior cause. Alterations are produced in the natural spirit by these causes together with those that are external, leading to moisture, dryness, *heat or cold,* and these are known as the cohesive causes of disease. For, in Athenaeus' view, the spirit, having penetrated the homoiomerous parts of the body, changes them through its own change and assimilates them to itself.

Often, he says, the cohesive cause is produced directly from the 4
immediate without an intermediary, though sometimes it comes through the medium of the prior cause. For example, when a man is affected by the heat of the sun, this produces a change in his natural spirit, which becomes hotter than it was before, and when he is affected by cold this spirit turns to cold. When these changes are slight, then the disease has not yet settled in the body. But when any part of the body has its natural composition distorted to such an extent that its actions are harmed, it has then been attacked by a disease produced through a defect in its composition. The cohesive cause of the disease is the spirit, which has gone too far towards either heat, cold, dryness or moisture. What the adherents of this school call prior causes are 5
the humours produced in our bodies when these are too hot, cold, *moist, or dry.* For they think that, with the passage of time, these alter the primary parts and assimilate them to their own condition, which

ومن قبل ذلك يدخل أيضا على أفعالها الضرر ويرون أنّ ممّا يجرى هذا المجرى ٦
سموم ذوات السموم مثل سمّ الكلب الكلِب وجميع الأدوية المضادّ طبعها لطبع
البدن من القتّالة وغيرها قالوا وبعض هذه السموم والأدوية ليست تفعل فى أبدان
الحيوان فعلا بيّن الرداءة إلّا بعد زمان طويل جدّا وذلك من قبل أنّ إحالتها
ليست تكون دفعة بل قليلا قليلا قالوا وكثرة الدم أيضا ربّما كانت سببا للأمراض

٣ وأمّا أنا فأقول انّ الأجسام الطبيعيّة إنّما تكوّنت من النار والأرض والماء
والهواء فإنّ بقراط قد كان قبل جميع الناس أورد البرهان عليه ولا فرق بين
أن تسمّى الاسطقسات من قبل جواهرها كما سمّيتها فى هذا الموضع فتقال
نار وماء وهواء وأرض وبين أن تسمّى من قبل كيفيّاتها فتقال رطب ويابس وحارّ
وبارد وأمّا أنّ الروح هو أوّلا يستحيل فى الأجسام الطبيعيّة ثمّ يحيل باستحالته
سائر الأجسام معه فلست أراه صوابا وذلك أنّ الروح ليس يبقى أصلا على ما كان ٢
عليه منذ أوّل الأمر متى وقع المزاج بينه وبين سائر الأجسام عند امتزاج الاسطقسات
الأربعة على الكلّيّة بعضها ببعض بل يحدث عن الأربعة جسم واحد خامس هو
غير كلّ واحد من تلك الأربعة ومثال ذلك المرهم المعروف بذى الأربعة الأدوية
فإنّا إذا عملنا هذا المرهم فخلطنا الشمع والزفت والراتينج والشحم فامتزجت ٣
بعضها ببعض على الكلّيّة فليس يبقى حينئذ واحد من هذه الأدوية بعد الخلط
على ما كان عليه قبله بل يحدث دواء واحد خامس غير كلّ واحد من الأدوية
الأربعة وذلك أنّه لا يكون عند الامتزاج ولا واحد منها خالصا على طبيعته حافظا
لها وكذلك يجرى الأمر فى الأجرام الصلدة فإنّك إن أخذت اقليميا وزاجا ٤
وزنجارا واسفيداجا فسحقتها سحقا ناعما حتّى تصير فى حدّ الغبار وخلطتها
بعضها ببعض لم يبق حينئذ كلّ واحد منها على ما كان عليه منذ أوّل الأمر

٤ فلذلك متى أحدث سبب من الأسباب التى من خارج فى الأعضاء
المتشابهة الأجزاء استحالة ما إمّا بإسخان وإمّا بتبريد وإمّا بتجفيف وإمّا بترطيب
فإنّ التغيير منه يقع بالمركّب بأسره إلّا أنّ الأولى أن يكون الذى يستحيل أوّلا
أرطب الأجسام كما نجد ذلك فى الأشياء التى من خارج متى وقع حمى الشمس على
الماء وعلى الحجارة بالسواء وأسرع استحالة من الماء الهواء فكذلك قلت أنا فى ٢
كثير من كتبى انّ القوّة التى ترد على البدن من خارج من شأنها أن تحيل أوّلا

2 ذوات] ذاوت Ms. 4 فعلا] فعالا Ms., *ut vid.* الرداءة] الردا Ms.
7 أورد *scripsi* : *vel* أوكد *vel* أدلى *legi potest* 18 عند *add.* S'

results in functional damage. Of this type, in their view, are the 6
poisons of venemous creatures, such as that of rabid dogs, and all
drugs, fatal and non-fatal, whose nature is opposed to that of the body.
Some of these poisons and drugs, they say, produce no obvious ill
effects in the animal body until a very long time has passed, because
the alteration they cause is not immediate but gradual. They also
claim that an abundance of blood is often a cause of disease.

3. As for my own view, I maintain that natural bodies are produced
simply from fire, *earth, water and air*, as Hippocrates first proved.
It makes no difference if you refer to the elements by their substances,
as I have done here, and talk of fire, water, air and earth, or if you call
them after their qualities and speak of *moist, dry, hot and cold.* As for
the theory that the spirit is the first thing to change in natural bodies,
its alteration then affecting the other things, this I do not consider to
be correct. For the spirit does not preserve its original state at all when 2
it is blended with other bodies in the total intermingling of the four
elements. Rather, from the four is produced a single fifth substance,
which is not identical with any one of its ingredients. An illustration
of that point is the unguent known as "The Quadruple". When we 3
make this we mix wax, *pitch, resin* and tallow and as these are com-
pletely intermingled none of them remains afterwards in its former
state. Rather, a single fifth medicament is produced which is not the
same as any of those four, since in the process of intermingling not
one of them preserves and maintains its nature intact. *The same is
true* of solids. When you take *litharge*, vitriol, verdigris and white lead, 4
pound them into a fine dust and then mix them with one another,
none of them remains in its original state [1].

4. When an external cause, then, produces some change in the
homoiomerous parts of the body, either by heating, cooling, drying
or moistening, this change will affect the whole compound, though
what changes first will most naturally be what contains most moisture.
That is what we find happening in externals, when the heat of the
sun strikes both water und rock equally, while air changes even more
rapidly than water. Thus it is that I have said in a number of my 2
works that the function of the force which impinges on the body

---

[1] The text followed by the translator is false, as this statement should be positive and not negative (see the Latin version and De elementis secundum Hippocratem I 413, 6sqq. K. = 1, 6sqq. Helmr.).

الجوهر الذى يسمّى جوهر الهواء والروح ثمّ تحيل ثانيا جوهر الرطوبات ثمّ حينئذ
تصل إلى جوهر الأجسام الأصليّة وتحيل أوّلا من هذا الجوهر أيضا السمين واللحم من
بعد ذلك تحيل الأجسام التى من جنس الأغشية والعصب ثمّ من بعد هذه الغضاريف
والعظام فإنّ فى الأفضية التى فى البدن جوهرا هوائيّا كما فيه جوهر رطب إلّا أنّه ٣
ليس لقائل أن يقول انّ الروح الذى فى الأجسام الأصليّة يستحيل قبل الرطوبات
وذلك أنّه ليس يلبث ويبقى الروح نفسه ولوكان يلبث لكان لعمرى سيستحيل ٤
بسرعة إذ كان على غاية التهيّؤ لقبول الاستحالة من الأشياء المسخنة والأشياء
المبرّدة والأشياء المرطّبة والأشياء المجفّفة كما نجد ذلك عيانا فى الهواء المحيط بنا
فإنّه قد يجب أن تكون الأجسام اللطيفة أول الأجسام استحالة وقد أصاب شيعة
اثيناوس ذلك فى اعتقادهم فإنّا نرى عيانا فى الحرّ الذى يكون عند طلوع الشعرى ٥
العبور أوّل ما يقبل حمى الشمس الهواء ثمّ بعد ذلك بقليل ما وقع عليه شعاع
الشمس من الرطوبات ماء كان أو غيره ثمّ بأخرة الأجرام الصلدة وأيضا فإنّ
الشمس إذا غربت فزال حميها كان الهواء أوّل ما يرجع إلى مزاجه الذى كان عليه
منذ أوّل الأمر ثمّ يتلوه فى ذلك الماء ثمّ بأخرة الحجارة وذلك أنّ ما كان سريع ٦
الاستحالة كان تغيّره إلى كلّ واحدة من الحالين المتضادّتين سريعا وما كان
بطىء الاستحالة فكما أنّ خروجه عن الأمر الطبيعىّ إنّما يكون فى زمان طويل
كذلك أيضا رجوعه إليه إنّما يكون فى زمان طويل فالحال فى أبدان الحيوان ٧
كالحال فى الأجرام التى لا أنفس لها من أنّ الجوهر الهوائىّ فيها أسرع ما فيها تغيّرا
والجوهر الرطب أبطأ منه وأبطأها كلّها جوهر الأعضاء الأصليّة حتّى أنّه متى نال ٨
عضوا من الأعضاء حرّ أو برد فأوّل ما يستحيل فيه طبيعة الهواء المحتبسة فى
الأفضية التى بين الأعضاء الأصليّة وفى كثير من البطون التى فى هذه الأعضاء ثمّ
بعدها طبيعة الرطوبة ثمّ من بعد ذلك طبيعة الأعضاء الأصليّة أنفسها التى هى
أعضاء أبداننا

٥ فإن أنت توهّمت أنّ هذه الجواهر الثلاثة قد خالطت بعضها بعضا على
الكلّيّة فليس يجوز لك حينئذ أن تقول انّ جوهر الهواء يستحيل أوّلا ثم جوهر
الرطوبة ثانيا ثمّ جوهر الأرض ثالثا وذلك أنّ امتزاج الأشياء بأسرها إنّما معناه ٢
أنّ كلّ واحد من الأشياء المختلطة قد استحال بأسره على الكلّيّة من قبل أنّه إن
كان كلّ واحد منها باقيا بعد الاختلاط على ما كان عليه قبل الاختلاط فإنّ ذلك

2 *ante* II من *fort.* و *addendum est* 9 *post* اللطيفة *fort.* الأجزاء *inserendum est*

externally is to change first what is known as the pneumatic and
spiritual substance and then, secondly, that of the moist elements.
Next it reaches the substance of the primary parts, where it alters
first the fat and the flesh, then what belongs to the class of membranes
and nerves and then the cartilages and bones. For in its interstices 3
the body contains a pneumatic substance, just as it contains a moist
one. No one, however, can say that in the primary parts the spirit
changes before the moist elements, for the spirit itself is not permanent.
If it were, it would certainly be quick to change, as it is preeminently 4
adapted to being altered by what is hot, cold, moist or dry, as can
plainly be seen in the air that surrounds us. For fine bodies must be
the first to change and the followers of Athenaeus are correct in that
part of their doctrine. So it is that in the heat when the Dog Star rises 5
we see that the first thing to be warmed by the sun is the air, then,
soon afterwards, whatever moisture is touched by its rays, whether
this be water or something else, while the last things to be affected
are the solids. Also when the sun sets and its heat diminishes the air
is the first thing to resume its original composition, followed in that
by the water and, finally, by the rocks. For whatever is quick to change 6
turns quickly to one or other of the two opposing states, but what is
slow to change takes a long time to leave its natural state but is also,
in the same way, slow to revert to it.

The position of animal bodies is like that of inanimate ones in that 7
the pneumatic substance is the quickest of their ingredients to change,
the moist being slower, and slowest of all is the substance of the
primary parts. So it is that, when some part of the body is affected 8
by heat or cold, the first thing to change in it is the nature of the air
confined in the interstices of the primary parts and in many of the
hollows that are to be found there. This is followed by what is naturally
moist and then by the nature of the primary parts themselves that
form our limbs.

5. However, if you imagine that these three substances have been
wholly intermingled, you cannot then say that the first to change is
the pneumatic, the second the moist and the third the earthy. For the 2
one meaning of total intermingling is that each ingredient has suffered
a complete change. If after they had been mixed these ingredients
were all to remain in their original state, that would imply that their

إنّما هو تقارب منها فى الوضع بأجزاء صغار لا امتزاج على الكلّيّة لكنّ هذا إنّما ٣
هو من عقد ابنادقليس وذلك أنّه كان يظنّ أنّ قوام الأجسام الطبيعيّة ليس هو
بامتزاج من الاسطقسات الأربعة بل باختلاط منها ولذلك صار رأيه فى هذا موافقا
لرأى شيعة افيقورس وديمقريطس فأمّا الفلاسفة أصحاب المظلّة فليس يقولون
بتقارب الوضع ولا ارسطوطاليس ولا من يقول بالروح من الأطبّاء إلّا أنّ ما قلته ٤
من ذلك إنّما قلته على طريق الاستظهار لأبيّن به أنّ ما يقوله أصحاب المظلّة
ينقض بعضه بعضا فإنّ القول بأنّ الاسطقسات يمازج بعضها بعضا على الكلّيّة
غير مطابق للقول بأنّ أوّل ما يقبل الاستحالة من الممتزج الروح لكنّه قد يحصل
للأطبّاء ما يحتاج إليه وإن لم يقل هذا القول وذلك أنّا قلنا ان العضو عند قبوله التأثّر ٥
يستحيل بأسره معا أو قلنا انّ الذى يستحيل منه أوّلا الروح ثمّ بتوسّط الروح
يستحيل سائر ما فيه فقد يلزمنا ضرورة أن يكون العلاج الذى نستعمله فيه واحدا
بعينه حتّى يدنى من الأعضاء التى قد بردت ما يسخنها ويدنى من الأعضاء التى
قد سخنت بأكثر من المقدار ما يبرّدها وكذلك يدنى من الأعضاء التى جفّت ما
يرطّبها ومن الأعضاء التى رطبت ما يجفّفها
٦ فأمّا من قال بأنّ المعرفة بالسطقسات ليس بالأطبّاء حاجة إليها أو قال
بأنّهم محتاجون إليها إلّا أنّه ممّن يؤثر رأيا ما غير رأى أصحاب المظلّة فليس
يتهيّأ أن يكون يعتقد أنّ لكلّ واحد من الأشياء الموجودة سببا ماسكا وقد نسمع ٢
كثيرا من الناس يقول انّ من القضايا الواجب قبولها من ذاتها لا برهان يقام
عليها أنّه ليس يمكن أن يكون جسم من الأجسام التى هى بحال من الأحوال
موجودا من غير أنّ يكون له سبب ماسك إلّا أنّهم يقولون انّ السبب الماسك ليس
هو موجودا فى الأجسام كلّها لكن فى الأجسام التى جوهرها جوهر يعسر انحلاله
وتفرّقه دون غيرها وممّا يجرى من الأجسام هذا المجرى حجر الصنام والصخر والعظام
والحديد وسائر ما أشبهها وقولهم هذا متناقض وذلك أنّه إن كان كلّ واحد من ٣
الأشياء الموجودة يحتاج إلى سبب يمسكه لا يمكن وجوده دونه فقد يجب لا محالة
أن يكون لذلك السبب أيضا إذا كان من الأشياء الموجودة سبب آخر يمسكه وأن
يكون لهذا أيضا سبب آخر يمسكه وأن يمرّ ذلك بلا نهاية إذ كان ليس يمكن
الوقوف عند واحد منها وإن قالوا انّ بعض الأشياء الموجودة متماسكة بذاتها ٤

3 موافق Ms. 9 *post* أنّا *fort.* إن *inserendum est* 13 حفّت S' : يبست Ms. 16 رأى *add.* S' 25 سبب] سببا Ms. 26 سبب] سببا Ms.

minute parts had simply been juxtaposed and not that they had been
totally intermingled. But this is just what Empedocles thought. For 3
he used to hold the view that natural bodies are produced not by an
intermixture of the four elements but by their combination and for
that reason on this point his theory coincides with that of the followers
of Epicurus and Democritus, whereas neither the Stoic philo-
sophers nor Aristotle talked of juxtaposition nor does the Animist
school of medicine. My remarks on that point were made only *by way* 4
of demonstration in order to show that the various sayings of the
Stoics are inconsistent. For to say that the elements are totally inter-
mingled does not coincide with the theory that the first part of the
compound to change is the spirit. Doctors, however, can get what they
need without committing themselves to this statement. For we can 5
say that, when something affects a part of the body, the whole of this
changes simultaneously, or we can say that the part of it that changes
first is the spirit and then, through the medium of this, the rest of its
elements change. But the remedies that we use must necessarily be
one and the same. To limbs that have been chilled we apply something
to heat them and to those that have been over-heated is given some-
thing that will chill them. Similarly we apply something to moisten
those that are dry and to dry those that are moist.

6. As for those who say that a knowledge of the elements is not
needed by doctors or who, while thinking that it is necessary, prefer
to follow a different theory to that of the Stoics, these people *cannot*
believe that everything that exists has a cohesive cause.

We hear a number of people say that amongst the propositions that 2
are *intrinsically acceptable without established proof* is that no body in
any state whatsoever can exist without having a cohesive cause. They
say, though, that this cause is not to be found in all bodies but, rather,
it exists in those whose substance it is particularly difficult to resolve
and dissipate, such as adamant, rock, *bones*, iron and other similar
things. But this remark of theirs is inconsistent in that, if every single 3
extant thing needs a cohesive cause without which it cannot exist,
that cause, as it is one of the existing things, must inevitably have
another cohesive cause itself which, in turn, must have yet another
and that will go on ad infinitum, nor can we stop at any one stage of
the process. But they may say that some existing things cohere through 4

وبعضها يحتاج فى ذلك إلى غيرها فقد يجب أن يكون ما كان جوهره سريعا إلى
التفرّق والانتشار حرىّ بأن يكوّن محتاجا إلى ما يمسكه   ينبغى أن يفهم هذا
الردّ على من قال بأنّ السبب الماسك إنّما هو الروح والروح عندهم جسم الناس
فأمّا ما كان جوهره مستحصفا متماسكا تماسكا قويّا فهو غير محتاج
إلى شىء من ذلك ولذلك صار الناس يضعون الخشب والحجارة والفضّة والذهب
والحديد والنحاس وسائر ما أشبهها من غير شىء يحصرها ويمسكها فأمّا الماء
والشراب والخلّ والعسل فيودعوها الحباب والخوابئ لأنّها ليست متماسكة بأنفسها
فليس منقاسا إذًا أن يكون الجسم الصلد يحتاج إلى ما يتماسك به وذلك أنّه إنّما ٥
صار صلدا صلبا لهذا المعنى بعينه أعنى لأنّه متماسك بنفسه وهذا أيضا ممّا يقدح
فى رأى أصحاب المظلّة أعنى أنّ جسما أرضيّا مثل حجر الصنام والصخر يتماسك
بجوهر من جنس الروح فإنّا نجد طبيعة الروح سريعة إلى التهبّى ونجد طبيعة الأرض
بطئة الانحلال وليس يمكن عندهم أن يخطر بالبال جوهر ما ولو كان فى غاية
الصغر مثل الهباء الذى يقول به ابيقورس متماسك بنفسه فضلا عن أن يكون
موجودا وذلك أنّه إمّا ألّا يكون للاسطقس الأرضىّ وجود أصلا إذ كان ليس ٦
يمكن أن يكون جزء من الأرض ولو كان فى غاية الصغر موجودا خلوّا من الجوهر
الروحانىّ وإمّا أن يكون قد يوجد من الأرض أجزاء وإن كانت فى غاية الصغر
مفردة بذاتها من غير أن تمازج الروح فهذه اثوما متماسكة لا محالة بذاتها إلّا
أنّ هذا القول إنّما قلناه كما قلنا ذلك القول الذى قبله على طريق الاستظهار
٧ وإنّى لأعجب من الأطبّاء الذين يقولون انّ المعرفة بالاسطقسات ليس يحتاج
إليها فى صناعة الطب كيف يسمّون أسبابا من الأسباب ماسكة فإنّا لسنا نجد شيئا
من الأشياء الموجودة يحتاج إلى أن يتماسك بجوهر آخر لكنّ كلّ واحد منها مكتف
بنفسه غير محتاج إلى غيره فى الوجود وإن استقصى الإنسان النظر كأنّه أن يجد كلًّ ٢
سبب فليس إنّما هو سبب لوجود ما أوّل بل لتكوّن والوجود   قال حنين
اليونانيّون يسمّون الجوهر والوجود باسم واحد   المتكوّن ليس هو أوّلا وذلك
أنّ التكوّن كأنّه طريق ما يؤدّى إلى الوجود ولذلك صارت الأشياء المتكوّنة فقط
يوجد لها أسباب للتكوّن وإن كان شىء من الأشياء غير متكوّن فلا أسباب له

2sq. ينبغى . . . . الناس *in marg.* Ms.   7 فيودعوها *sic*   14 وجودا] وجود Ms.
15 جزءا Ms.   16 من الأرض أجزاء : من الاض S¹ Ms.   17 اثوما] اذرة
suprascripsit S¹   23 لوجود] الوجود Ms.   أوّل] *fort.* أوّلا *corrigendum est*

their own nature, while others need something else to hold them. It follows that what has an easily dispersed substance is more likely to need a cohesive cause – *This refutation must be understood as applying to those who hold the cohesive cause to be the spirit, which, in their view, forms the human body*[1]. – ,while the need will not affect bodies whose substance is firmly compact. For that reason wood, rock, silver, gold, iron, copper and other similar things *are put down* without having anything to contain or hold them, while water, wine, vinegar and honey are stored in jars and containers, because they are not self-coherent. It is not logical, then, for solids to need a cohesive cause in that the 5 fact that they are solid and hard depends on this very quality, I mean that of self-coherence. This is also one of the criticisms that can be levelled against the Stoic theory, I mean that an earthy body, like adamant and rock, should be held together by a substance of the class of spirit. For we find that this latter is naturally quick to disperse while the dissolution of earth is a slow process. But according to these people it is impossible to imagine even the smallest substance, such as Epicurus' atoms, *as self-coherent let alone extant*. Either the element 6 of earth has no existence at all, since there can be no part of it, however small, without pneumatic substance, or else earth has parts, however small these may be, that are isolated and independent without any admixture of spirit, and these are necessarily self-cohesive atoms. This remark, like the one before, has been put forward *by way of demonstration*.

7. As for those doctors who say that a knowledge of the elements is unnecessary for medical science, I am surprised that they can call any cause cohesive. For no extant thing is found in need of another substance to hold it together. Rather, every one of them is self-sufficient and needs nothing else in its existence. If you make a thor- 2 ough examination, I think that you will find that every cause is the cause not of *primary* existence but of generation. For generated existence – *Ḥunain said: The Greeks use the same term for both substance and existence.* – does not come first, since the process of generation is as it were a path leading to existence. For that reason it is only *what has been generated that* has a cause which has produced it, and if there is anything that has not been generated, then it has no cause.

---

[1] Ḥunain is not mentioned by name in this note.

وافلاطن أيضا يقول فى كتابه المنسوب إلى طيماوس حين قال وكلّ ما يتكوّن ٣
فواجب ضرورة أن يتكوّن عن سبب من الأسباب وذلك أنّه محال من الجهات
كلّها أن يقع تكوّن بلا سبب لكنّ مـــا قد تكوّن وفرغ فواجب ضرورة أن
يكون إنّما تكوّن عن سبب موجود فأمّا ما هو موجود فليس يحتـــاج إلى سبب
٨ فمن أين ترى دخل الغلط على بعض الناس حتّى قالوا انّ لكلّ واحد من
الأشياء الموجودة سببا ماسكا أمّا أنا فأظنّ أنّ الغلط دخل عليهم من قبل أنّهم لم
يفرقوا بين الأشياء التى يقال فيها على الإطلاق والتحقيق انّها موجودة وبين الأشياء
التى ليس يقال ذلك فيها على التحقيق والإطلاق بل مع الاستثناء وذلك أنّ الأشياء ٢
التى لا تلبث أجزاؤها فليست تلك الأشياء موجودة على الإطلاق مثل الصوت والمشى
وكلّ فعل وانفعال وبالجملة كلّ حركة بنقلة كانت أو باستحالة فإنّه قد يظنّ أنّ
لهذه أسبابا ما ماسكة من لم يكن له خبرة صحيحة بطبيعتها حتّى يعلم أنّ
وجودهـــا انّمـــا هو فى التكـــوّن نفسه وليست موجودة على الإطلاق لأنّه ليس
يبقى جزء من أجزائها كما يبقى من كلّ واحد من الأشياء الموجودة وقد عرض مثل ٣
ذلك فى أمر النبض وذلك أنّهم لمّا رأوه يكون فى مدّة الحياة كلّها فى العروق
الضوارب والقلب ولا يفتر ظنّوا أنّه شىء من الأشياء الموجودة وليس النبض موجود
كالعروق الضوارب والقلب وسائر أعضاء البدن وذلك أنّ وجوده إنّما هو فى
التكوّن إذ كان ليس لجزء من أجزائه ثبات وقد يظنّ قوم أنّ لأجزائه ثباتا
من قبل أنّهم لا يقدرون على أن يفرقوا بأذهانهم بين المتكوّن وبين الموجود فإنّ ٤
المتكوّن يشبه الماء الجارى وأمّا الموجود فيشبه الماء القائم وكذلك يجرى الأمر فى
الأنهار وخاصّة إذا نظر الإنسان إليها من بعد فإنّه يتخيّل له ماء النهر كأنّه واقف
وليس شىء من أجزائه بالحقيقة ثابتا لكن من قبل أنّ الصورة العامّيّة للماء ثابتة
دائما فى الماء الجارى كثيرا ما يتخيّل لنا أنّ الماء واقف غير جار وكذلك أيضا النبض ٥
فإنّ ما منه قد تكوّن وفرغ فهو غير موجود وكذلك أيضا مًا هو مزمع بالتكوّن

1 *post* يقـول *fort.* ذلك *inserendum est* 4 موجود[1] *fort. omittendum est*
15 موجود *sic*

Plato makes the same point[1] in his book related to Timaeus. He 3
writes: "Everything that comes into existence must necessarily do so
as a result of some cause. That it should do so without a cause is
totally impossible." What has already come into existence and finished
with this process must have done so as the result of some existing
cause, but what is extant has no need of a cause.

8. From where do you think, then, that the mistake arose that has
caused some people to claim that every extant thing has a coherent
cause? My own view is that this is due to the fact that they drew no
distinction between what can be termed extant absolutely and accu-
rately and what cannot be so termed without qualification. For things 2
whose parts have no permanence have no absolute existence. Examples
of this are the voice and the process of walking, together with all
actions and passive experiences and, in general, all motion, whether
this is produced by locomotion or by change. These may be thought
to have cohesive causes, but only by those whose knowledge of their
natures is not sound enough to allow them to realise that they are
found only in the state of coming into being and have no absolute
existence. For no part of them has the permanence that is the quality
of existing things.

Something of this kind has happened with regard to the pulse. 3
People have seen it in the arteries and the heart, never failing through-
out the life span, and for that reason they have thought of it as some-
thing that exists. But, in fact, it is not extant in the same way as are
the arteries, the heart, and the other parts of the body. It is only to be
found in the state of coming into being, as no single part of it has any
permanence. Admittedly its parts may be thought of by some as per-
manent, but that is because these people are unable to make the
mental distinction between what comes into existence and what is
extant. For the former resembles running water and the latter water 4
that is still. You find the same thing in rivers, particularly when they
are seen *from a distance*. For then their water seems to be standing
still, though in fact no single part of it really is. But as the general
form of the water always remains fixed in the flowing stream, it often
seems to us that its water is still and not flowing. The same thing 5
applies to the pulse. What there is of it that has already come into
existence and been finished with does not exist nor does what is about

[1] Following the addition suggested in the apparatus.

والموجود منه إنّما هو ما يقع تحت الأصابع ما دام يقع تحتها على أنّ هذا أيضا
ليس هو موجودا على الإطلاق بل وجوده إنّما هو فى التكوّن وذلك أنّه ليس
يلبث جزء من أجزائه إذ كان كلّ واحد منها يبطل إذا تكوّن بل الأحوط أن
تقول حين يتكوّن فأمّا أسباب تكوّنه فقد بيّنّا أنّها ثلثة المنفعة التى بسببها ٦
احتيج إلى أن يكون والقوّة الحيوانيّة التى عنها تكوّن وجرم العروق الضوارب
والقلب الذى هو آلة له فإن آثرت أن تسمّى هذه الأسباب الأسباب الماسكة لتكوّن
النبض كما سمّيتها أنا فى مواضع كثيرة من كتابى فى النبض لا على التحقيق بل
على طريق الاستعارة لإيضاح القول وإيجازه فما بئس ما تصنع فى اللقب وقد يجرى ٧
هذا المجرى الرصاص فى بعض الأصنام التى تميل إلى قدّام فإنّ الصنم منها متى لم
يلتحم بدنه برجليه سقط على وجهه فإذا ألحم بالرصاص وقف منتصبا فإنّ
الميل فى الصنم من هذه بحسب طبيعته التى تخصّه باقٍ بعد اللحام على حاله إلّا
أنّ الرصاص يمنعه ويمسكه ويجذبه إلى ورائه فيجب من ذلك أن يكون ٨
الرصاص إنّما هو سبب لتكوّن ما لا لوجود على الإطلاق لكن لمّا كان هذا
المتكوّن يبقى ما بقى متشابه الحال صار يسبق إلى وهم من يراه أنّه أمر واحد مشار
إليه وليس ذلك أمرا مشارا إليه ولا هو وجود ما أصلا بل تكوّن فى موادٍّ كثيرة
مشار إليها عن سبب واحد ومثال ذلك ما يعرض لأصحاب التشنّج وذلك أنّ ٩
الحال الفاعلة لهذا العرض إذا بقيت فإنّ المتكوّن هو التشنّج والحال الباقية هى
سبب ماسك لتكوّنه وكذلك أيضا للسهر واختلاط الذهن والسبات والسعال وسوء ١٠
التنفّس وظلمة البصر وثقل السمع أسباب موجودة فى البدن فاعلة لهذه العلل
التى ذكرت وبعض الناس يسمّى الحالات أنفسها أمراضا ويقول انّ أصناف
ضرر الفعل هى أعراض لاحقة لهذه الحالات وبعضهم يسمّى أصناف ضرر
الأفعال أمراضا ويقول انّ أسبابها هى حالات الأبدان فأمّا أنّ منزلة الحالات ١١
بالقياس إلى أصناف الضرر منزلة الأسباب لها فأمر يقرّ به الجميع وكذلك أيضا قد
يقرّون بأنّ الغرض الأوّل المقصود إليه بالعلاج إنّما هو الحالات لا أصناف الضرر
وأمّا ما وقع فيه الاختلاف فإنّما هو فى اللقب لكنّه قد يلزم أهل الفرقة الأولى أعنى ١٢
الذين يسمّون حالات الأبدان أمراضا ألّا يقولوا انّ هاهنا سببا ماسكا فى

5 تكوّن] *fort.* يتكوّن *legendum est* 15 وجودا Ms. 17 الحال[II] *ex* الحل, *ut vid.*, S¹

to come into existence. In fact, its only extant part is what lies beneath
the fingers at the moment that it actually does so, though even this
has no absolute existence but one that is found only in generation.
For no single one of its parts is permanent, but each one passes away
when once it *has come into being* or, put more comprehensively, at the
time when it *comes into being*. As for the causes of its generation, these 6
I have shown to be three in number, that is, the useful purpose because
of which we need this, the animal force from which it is generated and
the structure of the arteries and of the heart which serves as an instru-
ment for it. There is no harm in calling these things, if you choose,
cohesive causes for the generation of the pulse, as I myself have often
done for clarity and conciseness in my book "On the Pulse", though
this is not an actual but, rather, a metaphorical use of terms. A parallel 7
here is the use of lead in some statues that lean forwards. Where the
body of one of these statues is not firmly attached to its feet, it will
fall on its face, but if it is secured with lead it will stand upright. For,
though the natural inclination peculiar to it will still remain as it was,
the lead will check, hold, and draw it backwards. It follows that the 8
lead is a cause only of some form of generation and not of absolute
existence. But since what is generated here remains for its whole span
in a self-consistent state, those who see it first imagine that it is a
single *determinate* thing, though it is neither, in fact, *determinate* nor
any form of *existence* at all, but rather generation that takes place in a
quantity of *determinate* matter through a single *cause*.

Now look, as an example, at what happens to paralytics. While 9
the condition that produces this symptom remains, what is generated
is the convulsion, and the persisting condition is the cohesive cause of
its generation. Similarly, for insomnia, mental disorder, *stupor*, 10
coughing, defective respiration, dulled eyesight and heaviness of
hearing there are efficient causes existing in the body. Some call the
conditions themselves diseases and hold that the types of functional
injury are symptoms associated with them. *Others call the types of
functional injury diseases* and class the bodily conditions as their
causes. It is a matter of general agreement that the relationship of the 11
conditions to the types of injury is that of cause and effect and it is
also agreed that what we should aim at first in our cure is the condition
and not the various injuries. Where disagreement does occur, it centres
simply on nomenclature. It follows that the adherents of the first 12
school, I mean those who call bodily conditions diseases, should not

الأمراض أصلا ويلزم أهل الفرقة الأخرى ما قلته قبيل أن يكونوا يستعملون على
طريق الاستعارة اسم السبب الماسك على الحالات إذ كان ضرر الأفعال إنّما
يحدث عنها

٩ فهذا هو القول على طريق الرسم فى الأسباب الماسكة فى الأبدان السقيمة
وأمّا فى الأبدان السليمة فما قلته آنفا وهو أنّه إن كان العضو متشابه الأجزاء فليس لنا
أن نقول انّ له سببا ماسكا وإن كان آليّا مركّبا فلنا أن نقول ذلك فى الأشياء التى
تصل وتقرن الجواهر الأول البسيطة التى منها تركّب وأمّا من كان من أصحاب ٢
المظلّة فقد قلت انّه يقول بأنّ لهذه أيضا الأجسام الأول المتشابهة الأجزاء سببا
ماسكا وهو جوهر الروح إلّا أنّه قد يجب على جميع الناس فضلا عن أصحاب
المظلّة الإقرار بما قلته آنفا من أنّ الأجسام الثوانى المركّبة تجرى مجرى الأجسام التى
يؤلّفها الصنّاع فى أنّ لها أسبابا ماسكة فكما أنّا نجد تأليف الكراسى والأسرّة ٣
والدرج والسفن والبيوت إنّما يحفظه ويبقيه الطين والجبسين والكلس والضبّات
والمسامير والمداخلة وسائر ما أشبهها كذلك الذى يبقى تأليف البدن الرباطات
والأوتار واللحم والغضاريف ومن العظام ما يعسر انحلال تركيبه لأسباب غير هذه
مثل العظام التى قد نجدها قد ألّف بعضها مع بعض على طريق المداخلة أو على
طريق الغرز أو على طريق الشأن أو على طريق المطابقة وقد يقول بأنّ الأجسام ٤
أيضا المتشابهة الأجزاء أنفسها التى هى على طبيعتها الذاتيّة لها مركّبة هذا التركيب
الذين يقولون بالاسطقسات التى يلقّبها اسقليبيادس بغير المؤتلفة ويلقّبها غيره بالتى
فى غاية الصغر ويلقّبها شيعة ابيقورس خاصّة بالأجزاء التى لا تتجزّأ وذلك أنّهم ٥
يرون أنّ الأجسام الطبيعيّة إنّما تكون بأنّ هذه تختلط وتتركّب ضربا من
التركيب وأنّ الأجسام الأول البسيطة أنفسها التى هى اسطقسات الأجسام المحسوسة
ليس لها سبب ماسك أصلا فأمّا ما تركّب منها فإنّ التركيب نفسه الذى يكون
منها عند اختلاطها هو سبب ماسك للمركّب فأمّا من قال انّ حمى الرأس من ٦
الشمس هو سبب ماسك للسخونة الحادثة فى الرأس وانّ الشقّ هو سبب ماسك
للجرح فإنّما أتى من قبل أنّه لم يشعر بأنّه فى هذا القول إنّما هو ذا يعبّر على
معنى واحد بعينه بأسماء مختلفة وذلك أنّ حمى الرأس من الشمس ليس هو
شيئا غير السخونة الحادثة فى الرأس عن شعاع الشمس وكذلك ليس الجرح

13 والمدا لمة *sic* : *fort. omittendum est*   18 الذين] الذى Ms.

talk of there being here a cohesive cause in disease at all, while the followers of the other school, as I said shortly before, must apply the term metaphorically to the conditions, since it is from them that the functional injuries are produced.

9. This account sketches the position of the cohesive cause in the
diseased body. In the healthy body this position is, as I said before,
that, if a part is homoiomerous, it cannot be said to have a cohesive
cause. But where it is an organic compound, that term can be used of
what connects and combines the primary simple substances of which
it is compounded. As for the Stoics, I have said that they claim these 2
primary homoiomerous substances also to have a cohesive cause in the
pneumatic essence. But not only the Stoics, but everyone else as well
must admit the proposition that I stated earlier. This was that second-
ary compound bodies resemble those constructed by craftsmen in that
they do have cohesive causes. We find that the composition of *chairs*, 3
bedsteads, *ladders*, ships and houses is guarded and preserved by clay,
gypsum, lime, nails, *pegs*, *wedges* and other similar things, and in the
same way the composition of the body is preserved by ligaments,
tendons, flesh and cartilages. There are also some bones whose junction
is hard to part for other reasons, such as those that are found to be
connected by inter-penetration, grafting, suturing, or by the apposition
of their surfaces. As for the homoiomeries themselves which are in 4
their natural and peculiar state, it may be said of them also that they
are compounded in this way by those who hold to the theory of the
elements which Asclepiades calls "disunited", others "minute",
and the Epicureans, in particular, "the indivisible particles". For 5
they think that natural bodies come into being simply through some
form of intermingling on the part of these things, while the primary
and simple bodies themselves, which serve as elements for the sen-
sibles, have no cohesive cause at all. As for what is compounded from
them, it is the composition itself resulting from their intermingling
that is the cohesive cause of the compound.

There are those who say that the heating of the head by the sun is 6
the cohesive cause of the warmth that results in it and that the cut is
the cohesive cause of the wound. But they only do this because they
do not realise that in saying this they are simply expressing the same
idea in different words. For the heating of the head by the sun implies
nothing more than warmth being produced in it by the sun's rays, nor

شيئا سوى الشقّ الذى يكون فى اللحم فإنّ لفظة الشقّ تدلّ على معنى جنسىّ ٧
يحدث فى الأجسام المتّصلة كلّها وذلك أنّا نسمّى تفرّق اتّصال هذه الأجسام
شقّا وأمّا الجرح والكسر والفسخ والهتك فيشتمل كلّ واحد منها فى دلالته على
معنيين أحدهما على الشقّ نفسه والآخر على الجسم الذى يحدث فيه وذلك أنّ
الشقّ إن كان حدوثه فى الجلد أو فيه وفى اللحم الذى من ورائه
سمّيت هذه العلّة جرحا وإن كان حدوثه فى عضلة سمّى ذلك فسخا وإن كان
حدوثه فى عظم سمّى ذلك المرض كسرا وإن كان حدوثه فى عضو عصبىّ سمّى
ذلك هتكا

١٠ فأمّا هذه العلل فإنّ حالات الأعضاء فيها ظاهرة بيّنة وأمّا ذات
الجنب وذات الرئة وزلق الأمعاء والسرسام البارد والسرسام الحارّ فإنّ
حالات الأعضاء فيه خفيّة لكنّ الأعراض الحادثة عنها واضحة وذلك أنّا نجد
المرضى عيانا يعرض لهم فيها اختلاط الذهن والسهر والألم وسوء التنفّس والسعال
والنفض الخارج عن الطبيعة فمن قال انّ حالات الأبدان هى أسباب ماسكة ٢
لحدوث هذه الأعراض كان قوله أحوط من قول من قال على الإطلاق انّ حالات
الأبدان هى أسباب ماسكة لهذه الأعراض من غير أن يستثنى فيقول لحدوث هذه
الأعراض أو تكوّنها فإنّ قول من قال انّ حالات الأبدان أسباب ماسكة لحدوث ٣
الأعراض أو تكوّنها قول لازم للقياس فأمّا القول بأنّها أسباب للأعراض التى
تحدث أنفسها فغير واجب اللّهمّ إلاّ أن يشاء إنسان أن يستعمل هذه
العبارة على طريق الاستعارة كما قلت وأمّا أصحاب التجربة فإنّهم يسمّون ما ٤
وصلوا إلى معرفته بالحواسّ من الأشياء التى تعرض لنا ونحن مرضى عوارض
وأعراضا وذلك لازم لمذهبهم وما كان من ذلك قد رآه قوم بعد قوم منهم مرارا
كثيرة يكون أوّل حدوثه وتزيّده بعد ومنتهاه وانحطاطه معا سمّوه مرضا وعلّة
واقتران فإنّ اسم الاقتران يدلّ عندهم على اجتماع ما لأعراض يكون حدوثها
وتزايدها وانحلالها معا ومن عادتهم أن يسمّوا ما كان كذلك من الأعراض دلائل ٥
أيضا وبالحقيقة أنّها دلائل لهيآت البدن التى هى غير ظاهرة وهى التى يسمّونها هم
أسبابا للأعراض الظاهرة إلاّ أنّهم ليس يعتقدون بالحقيقة أنّها تدلّ على الحالات

11 فيه] فيها *correxerit* Strohmaier 13 والنفض] والنفث *sec. Lat. emendaverit* Strohmaier 22 أوّل] *fort.* أوّلا *corrigendum est* 23 واقتران] واقران Ms., *ut vid.* 24 وانحلاها Ms. 25 التى[I] *add.* S¹

is the wound anything except the cut in the flesh. For the word "cut" 7
refers generically to what affects all connected bodies, to whose dis-
junction we give this name. As for the terms wound, fracture, severing
and tear, each contains an indication of two notions, one being that
of the cut itself and the other that of the body in which it occurs. For
if it affects the skin, or the skin and the flesh behind it, then the injury
is known as a wound. If it occurs in a muscle, it is called a severing;
if in a bone, a fracture, and if it affects a nerve tissue, it is known as
a tear.

10. In these injuries the condition of the affected parts is clearly visible. But in the case of pleurisy, pneumonia, lientery, lethargy and inflammation of the brain the state of the parts concerned is obscure and it is the *symptoms* resulting from these states that can be seen. For there we see plainly enough that the patients are affected by mental disorder, insomnia, pain, defective respiration, coughing and unnatural *feverish shivering*[1].

If you say, then, that bodily conditions are the cohesive causes of 2
the production of these symptoms, this is fuller than saying abso-
lutely that such conditions are the cohesive causes of the symptoms,
without adding as a qualification "of their production or generation".
For though it is analogically sound to say that these conditions are 3
cohesive causes of their production or generation, it is not logical to
say that they are the causes of the symptoms themselves that are thus
produced, unless, as I have said, you want to use this expression meta-
phorically. As for the Empiricists, in accordance with their doctrine, 4
of the things that affect us when we are ill, they call what can be re-
cognised by the senses fits and symptoms. In the same context, what
succeeding generations of them have often observed as being first
produced, then having an increase, followed together by a climax and
a decline, they call disease, sickness or syndrome – a term that they
apply to an accumulation of symptoms that occur, increase and are
resolved together. They are also in the habit of calling symptoms of 5
this kind signs, as they do, in fact, indicate the obscure states of the
body, which they call the causes of the obvious *states*. However, they
cannot really believe that these things do indicate states, for they

[1] Or, following the conjecture, "discharge".

وذلك أنّهم ليس يعترفون أصلا بالمعرفة التى تقع على طريق الاستدلال بالظاهر على
الخفىّ ولست أدرى كيف صار الجميع بأخرة إلى أن يسمّوا هذه المعرفة إدراكا فإنّ ٦
القول المستفيض الذى إحدى قضيّتيه وهى الأولى أنّه متى كانت دلائل كذا
فأسبابها كذا والقضيّة الثانية متى كانت أسباب كذا فالعلاج كذا ليس بهواه
أصحاب التجربة لكنّهم أخذوا ما اتّفق عليه من ذلك أصحاب القياس وألزموا
أنفسهم القول بالأسباب كأنّه أمر مطابق لقولهم فأمّا أصحاب القياس فإنّه وقع ٧
بينهم أنفسهم اختلاف لا يحصل منه انتفاع فى أعمال الطبّ فقال بعضهم كما
قلت انّ الأمراض هى حالات الأبدان وقال بعضهم انّ الأمراض هى أصناف
الضرر الحادثة عنها فى الأفعال وإذ كان الفريقان متّفقين على أنّ العلاج إنّما ٨
يستخرج من قبل الحالات على طريق الاستدلال فقد يسهل عليك أن تعلم أنّ
هذا الخلاف إنّما هو فى باب من أبواب المنطق وأنّه ليس ينفعنا ولا يضرّنا فى
أعمال الطبّ وذلك أنّك وإن سمّيت حالات البدن أمراضا فإنّك تفعل مثل ما
يفعل من يسمّيها أسبابا للأمراض من أنّك إنّما تستخرج العلاج منها على طريق
الاستدلال كما يستخرجه ذاك وتعدّ منه مثل ما يعدّه وتستعمله كما يستعمله

14 *in fine add.* تمت مقالة جالينوس فى الاسباب الماسكة وكتب خلف بن ابى الربيع الاندلسى لنفسه والحمد لله ذى القدرة التامة والنعمة العامة وصلواته على محمد رسوله واله عارضها بالاصل المنسوخ منه فصح بحسب الطاقة Ms.

refuse to acknowledge any cognition based on indications given about
what is obscure by what is obvious. Nor do I know how they all
eventually come to call this type of cognition comprehension. The 6
syllogism, *in full*, has as the first of its premises the statement that,
when the signs are such the causes are such, and the second premise
is that, when the causes are such the cure is such. But the Empiricists
do not approve of this. Rather, they have taken up here a point on
which the Dogmatists are agreed *and they have adopted the theory of
causes as though it was something that fitted in with their views.* The 7
Dogmatists themselves differ, but on a point from which there is no
benefit to be derived for the practice of medicine. For some hold, as
I said, that diseases are bodily states and others that they are the
types of functional injury that result from these states. But both 8
schools of thought are agreed that cures are to be deduced indicatively
from conditions, and you can readily understand, then, that the
difference is one that concerns logic and is of no help or hindrance in
medical practice. For if you call bodily conditions diseases, you will
still act in the same way as the man who calls them causes of disease,
and you will produce your cure only by the indications given, as he
does, *make the preparations that he makes and employ them as he does.*

CONSPECTVS SIGLORVM

A = Aya Sofya 3631
B = Aya Sofya 3590
B^1 = correctiones primae manus eiusdem codicis

كتاب جالينوس
فى تدبير الأمراض الحادّة على رأى بقراط

GALEN'S WORK ON REGIMEN IN ACUTE DISEASES IN ACCORDANCE WITH THE THEORIES OF HIPPOCRATES

كتاب جالينوس فى تدبير الأمراض الحادّة على رأى بقراط

١ قال إنّة لو لم يكن أحد تقدّمنى إلى معرفة الحقّ من أمر تدبير بقراط للأمراض
الحادّة لقد كنت سارعت إلى ما أمرتنى به من الكتاب أيّها الشّجاع بقطرينس
لكن لمّا كان كثير ممّن تقدّمنى قد فسّر الكتاب الذى وصف فيه بقراط أمر ذلك
التدبير تفسيرا صالحا رأيت أنّ الأجود أن أصف لك بلسانى فى وقت ما سألتنى
من ذلك مذهب بقراط فى تدبير أصحاب الأمراض الحادّة وذلك أنّى رأيت أنّ
الكلام من الحىّ أبلغ لك فى إفهامك ما قصدت إليه من الكلام الذى تقرأه بدءا فى
كتاب فإن بدا لك أن تسأل منه عن شىء قد غمض عليك أو قد ظننت أنّه لم يجر
القول فيه على الصواب لم تجد فيه جوابا لما قد تسأل عنه فلمّا رأيتك قد ألححت علىّ ٢
بالتقدّم إلىّ بأن يكون ما أصفه لك من أمر ذلك التدبير فى كتاب دون المخاطبة رأيت
أنّ أوّل ما ينبغى لك أن تعلمه وينبغى لى أن أعلّمك إيّاه أنّك إن كنت إنّما
تقصد إلى أن تعلم مذهب بقراط كلّه فى ذلك التدبير على الاستقصاء فالرأى
لك أن تقرأ فى الكتب التى وضعها كثير من الأطبّاء ممّن تقدّم ففسّر فيها
طريق بقراط فى تدبير الأمراض الحادّة وإن كنت إنّما تقصد إلى أن تعرف
جمل ذلك فقط فإنّى مجيبك إلى ما سألت لكنّه قد ينبغى لك أن تعلم أنّ بيان
المعنى فى ذلك ينقص بحسب نقصان الكلام الذى يعبّر به عنه عن المقدار المعتدل
وأنّ الأمرين جميعا كانا يستجريـان منّى عن غير إرادة ان أنا أجبتك إلى ما ٣
سألت أعنى كتابى فى معنى ليس عندى فيه زيادة على ما تقدّم فوصف فيه
وأكثر من ذلك أيضا التماسى أن أعبّر عن معنى لا يكاد الكلام الواسع يأتى
على شرحه وإيضاحه إلّا بكدّ بإيجاز واختصار لم أزل فى كلّ مرّة كنت تقتضينى

1 *ante titulum add.* بسم الله الرحمن الرحيم AB   5 رأيت أنّ] كان B
7 بدءا *om.* B   9 قد[I] *om.* A   10 فى *om.* A   11 *ante* لى *add. et del.* لك A
إيّاه *om.* A   13 وضعها] وصفها B   14 طرق B   17 وأنّ] فلان B

GALEN'S WORK ON REGIMEN IN ACUTE DISEASES IN ACCORDANCE WITH THE THEORIES OF HIPPOCRATES

1. If no one before me had understood how Hippocrates really treated acute diseases, my brave[1] Victorinus[2], I would have been quick to write about it, as you ordered me. However, since many of my predecessors have written sound commentaries on the work in which Hippocrates deals with that treatment for us, I thought that the best thing for me to do would be to explain his views on the subject verbally, when you asked me about this. For I considered that viva voce explanation would be more effective in making you understand what you wanted to know than an account that you would begin by reading in a book. For there, if it occurred to you to ask about anything which you found obscure or which you thought was wrongly stated, you would not be able to find an answer to your questions.

I saw, however, that you persisted in demanding that my account 2
of that treatment should be written and not oral and so I thought that the first point for you to learn and the first thing I should tell you is this. If what you want to do is to reach a thorough understanding of the whole of Hippocrates' doctrine on regimen in acute diseases, you had better study the books written by a number of other doctors in which this has already been explained. But if all you want is a summary, I would agree to your request, though you should realise that, as the explanatory account in that case would be disproportionately short, the explanation would be similarly defective.

Of the alternatives here, neither would I follow willingly. I do not 3
wish to agree to a request by you to write an account of something where I can add nothing to the explanations that have already been given. Still less do I wish to be asked to write a concise explanation of something which, except with difficulty, it is hardly possible to explain clearly in an expanded commentary. So I continued to put you off

---

[1] κράτιστε (?) (cf. XIX 8, 4 K. = Scr. min. II 91, 1).

[2] Βίκτωρι τῷ ʽΡώμης ἐπάρχῳ CMG V 9, 1 p. 265, 22.

ما سألت أدافعك وأماطلك به فإذ قد وقعت مدّة فيما كنت أدافع به لا بإرادتى لكن مكرها فإنّى جاعل افتتاح كلامى قولا قاله بقراط وهو أنّه قال انّه متى بلغ ٤ المرض منتهاه فيجب ضرورة أن يستعمل فيه التدبير الذى هو فى الغاية من اللطافة ومن الأمراض ما يبلغ منتهاه فى اليوم الثانى ومنها فى اليوم الثالث ومنها فى اليوم الرابع ومنها بالجملة فى أحد الأيّام التى بعد هذه فما كان من الأمراض لا يأتى عليه بعد مبتدأه مدّة طويلة حتّى يبلغ منتهاه فليس يغذو فيه المريض بتّة حتّى ينضج المرض إلّا أن يعرض عارض من الأعراض التى تهدّ القوّة فتضطرّ إلى أن يغذو المريض فأمّا الأمراض التى لا تبلغ منتهاها إلّا بعد مدّة طويلة فإنّ ٥ بقراط يرى أنّه إن لم يغذ المريض بتّة فيها قبل وقت منتهى مرضه سقطت قوّته وينبغى فى هذه الأمراض أن يتفكّر الطبيب منذ أوّل المرض وينظر هل يكتفى المريض بأن يقتصر بـه على السكنجبين أو ماء العسل فيسقى من أحدهما شيئا فى كلّ يوم إلى وقت منتهى المرض أم هل يحتاج أن يسقى مع ذلك ماء كشك الشعير أم ليس يكتفى بذلك أيضا دون أن يكون مع مـاء كشك الشعير شىء من ثفله فأىّ هذه الأشياء رآه أجود استعمله منذ أوّل المرض إلّا أن يكون المريض ٦ قريب العهد بالأكل فجوفه ملآن من الطعام أو هو محتاج إلى فصد أو إلى إسهال أو إلى علاج بحقنة أو بشيافة فإنّه يأمر إذا كانت تلك حال المريض أن يستعمل أوّلا كلّ واحد من هذه الأشياء التى ذكرت ثمّ يغذو المريض ويأمر أيضا أن يمسك عن الغذاء فى أوقات نوائب الحمّى

٢ فهذه هى جملة قوله وأصوله الأول وأمّا ما بعد ذلك ممّا يتلو ما ذكرنا فهو ما أصف أنزل أنّ حال المريض فى مرضه حال يأتيه معها البحران إمّا فى اليوم الرابع وإمّا فى اليوم الخامس وافهم عنّى فى كلامى هذا من قولى بحران كلّ ميل ذى قدر يكون إلى الحال التى هى أجود والبحث عن هذا الميل هل يكون فى وقت

1 أدافع] أدفع B   2 قال انّه *om.* B   6 *post* يبلغ *add.* الى B   8 لا *om.* B
9 منتهى *om.* B   10 ينبغى] ىسى *ut vid.* B   12 ماء *om.* B
15 وجوفه ممتلئ B   16 يأمر] يامن B   17 كلّ واحد] واحدا B
19 جمل B

and to temporise every time you demanded that I grant your request. But now after a period of postponement, not of my will but under pressure, I make my beginning with a quotation from **Hippocrates**.
Hippocrates says that when the disease reaches its climax we must 4
necessarily employ the lightest regimen[1]. Some diseases reach their climax on the second day, others on the third, others on the fourth and others, generally speaking, on one of the following days. When no long time passes from the start of the disease until its climax, the patient is given no food at all until his disease matures, unless some accidental complication occurs which impairs his strength and makes
it necessary to feed him. As for the cases where the climax only comes 5
after a long time, **Hippocrates'** opinion is that, if the patient is not fed at all before it, his strength will decline[2]. Here the doctor must consider from the start of the disease the question of whether it is enough for him to be kept on oxymel or honey water and to be given one of the two to drink every day until his climax, or whether he needs to be supplied with some barley gruel as well. It may be that not even this will be enough without the addition of some barley groats to-
gether with the gruel. Whichever of these is considered most suitable 6
should be used from the start of the disease, except in cases where the patient has recently eaten and his stomach is full of food, or where he requires bleeding, a purge, a clyster or a suppository[3]. For there **Hippocrates** recommends that the various remedies mentioned should first be applied and that the patient should be fed afterwards. He also recommends that the patient should be kept from food at the recurrent crises of his fever[4].

2. This, then, is the sum of his remarks and these are his first principles. The next point to be made, following on from what we have said, is as follows. Suppose that the state of the patient's disease is such that the crisis occurs either on the fourth or on the fifth day. You must understand, by the way, that when I say crisis here, I mean any measurable turn for the better[5]. To investigate whether this takes

---

[1] Aphor. I 8 *ὁκόταν δὲ ἀκμάζῃ τὸ νούσημα, τότε λεπτοτάτῃ διαίτῃ ἀναγκαῖον χρέεσθαι.* (IV 464, 1 sq. L.).

[2] Cf. Aphor. I 4 (IV 460,7–462, 2 L.).

[3] *φλεβοτομία, κάθαρσις, βάλανος, κλυστήρ* CMG V 9, 1 p. 134, 7 sq.

[4] Aphor. I 11 *ἐν δὲ τοῖσι παροξυσμοῖσιν ὑποστέλλεσθαι χρή·* (IV 464, 11 L.).

[5] *κρίσιν νῦν εἴρηκεν ἤτοι τὴν τελείαν λύσιν τοῦ νοσήματος ἢ τὴν εἰς τοσοῦτον ἀξιόλογον μεταβολήν* CMG V 9, 1 p. 145, 1 sq.

منتهى المرض فقط أو قد يكون كثيرا من قبل منتهاه بقليل يحتاج فيه إلى كلام
كثير لا يتّصل بغرضنا فى كتابنا هذا فأنا تارك البحث عن ذلك ونتنزل أنّ المريض ٢
الذى حاله الحال التى يأتيه البحران معها فى الرابع أو فى الخامس فى المثل معه من
القوّة ما يحتمل أن يبقى من غير أن يغتذى بتّة إلى أن يأتيه البحران فأقول انّ المريض
الذى هذه حاله ليس يسقيه بقراط لا ماء الشعير ولا ماء العسل ولا اسكنجبين
لكنّه يتركه خاويا خاليا إلى أن يجوز منتهى مرضه فإن كانت قوّة المريض محتاجة
إلى بعض الرفد فهو يرى أنّ ذلك المريض يكتفى بماء العسل وكذلك أيضا متى كان
المريض يتوقّع له البحران فى السابع وقوّته قويّة فإنّه يرى أنّه يكتفى بماء العسل
فأمّا السكنجبين فقد يسقيه بعض المرضى على طريق الدواء لا طريق الغذاء
وكذلك قد يسقى كثيرا من المرضى ماء العسل وماء الشعير أيضا على هذا الطريق إلّا ٣
أنّك ليس تحبّ أن تعلم متى يحتاج إلى هذه الأشياء على طريق الدواء لكنّ
قصدك فى مسئلتك إنّما كان كما قد علمت لأن تعلم هل كان بقراط يغذو
أصحاب الأمراض الحادّة فى كلّ يوم وقلت انّ بعض الأطبّاء ذكر لك ذلك
واعلم وليعلم المتطبّب الذى ذكر لك ما ذكر أنّ بقراط كثيرا ما يمنع المريض من ماء
الشعير ومن كلّ طعام غيره ويقتصر به على ماء العسل فقط وكثيرا ما يمنع أيضا من
ماء العسل ويقتصر بالمريض على إسقائه الماء فقط فإذا علم أنّ البحران يتأخّر ٤
إلى اليوم التاسع أو الحادى عشر أو الرابع عشر وأنّ قوّة المريض لا تحتمل أن
تبقى من غير غذاء غذا المريض منذ أوّل مرضه بكشك الشعير فقط من غير أن
ينيله معه غذاء غيره بتّة ولا يزيده على أن يحسيه من كشك الشعير شيئا فى كلّ
يوم خلا الأيّام التى يكون فيها للحمّى نوبة قويّة أو الأيّام التى يكون الجوف
فيها ممتلئا طعاما أو ثفل طعام فإنّه فى تلك الأيّام أيضا لا يغذو كما قلت قبيل
وذلك أنّه متى كان فى الجوف ثفل من طعام فينبغى أن يستفرغ أوّلا وإذا كان فى

2 تارك البحث [اولى بالبحث B   منزل B   3 التى [الذى A
المثل [الميل B   6 وان B   7 فهو *om.* A   8 البحران [بحران B
11 تحبّ [تجب B   13 لك *om.* B   14 واعلم [فاعام B   15 على *bis scr.* B
21 فيها ممتلئا [مملوءا فيها B   الأيّام *om.* A   قبيل [قبل B

place only at the climax of the illness or whether it may often happen a little before requires a long discussion which is not relevant to the object of my present work and I shall accordingly leave aside any enquiry into the point. Let us suppose, then, by way of example that 2
the condition of our patient is such that the crisis will occur either on the fourth or fifth day and that he has strength enough to last until then without being fed at all. I say that Hippocrates would not give anyone in this condition either barley water, honey water or oxymel to drink. Rather, he would leave him unfed and empty until the climax of his illness was past. But if his strength needs some sustaining, Hippocrates thinks that he should content himself with honey water[1], and the same treatment applies in cases where the crisis is expected on the seventh day and the patient is strong, as honey water is considered to be enough for him. As for oxymel, it is given to some by way of medicine, not by way of food, and this is done in the case of many patients with honey water and barley water also.

However, you do not want to know when these things are needed 3
medicinally, but rather, as I am aware, the purpose of your questions was simply to learn whether Hippocrates feeds every day those who are suffering from acute diseases. For you say that some doctor has told you that he does. But you must know, and so must the doctor who told you this, that Hippocrates frequently denies a patient barley water, together with every other form of food, and confines him to honey water alone. Often he keeps him from this as well and confines him solely to drinking water.

It may be, though, that you know that the crisis of the disease will 4
be postponed till the ninth, eleventh or fourteenth day and that the patient will not be strong enough to remain without being fed. Hippocrates then feeds him from the start of his illness on barley gruel alone[2], without giving him any other kind of food at all. So he is given no more than a daily portion of this gruel, except on days when he suffers from violent fits of fever or when his belly is full either of food or of its sediment. For then also he is not fed at all, as I said shortly before. That is because, when there is food sediment in the belly, it must first be evacuated, and when there is food in the stomach, it

[1] Cf. De diaet. in morb. acut., I 137, 3 Kw.

[2] *εἰ δ' εἰς τὴν ἐνάτην ἢ τεσσαρεσκαιδεκάτην ἢ εἰκοστὴν ἐμπίπτειν μέλλει τὸ νόσημα, χυλῷ πτισάνης ἐξ ἀρχῆς ἐπ' αὐτοῦ χρώμεθα.* CMG V 9, 1 p. 283, 20–22.

المعدة طعام فينبغى أن يترك حتّى ينحدر وكذلك أيضا متى كان المريض يحتاج
إلى أن يفصد أو يسهل فليس يغذوه حتّى يستعمل ما يحتاج إلى استعماله من
ذلك فأنزل أنّ المريض الذى يتوقّع له البحران فى اليوم التاسع أو الحادى عشر ٥
أو الرابع عشر ليس يحتاج إلى شىء من هذه الأشياء التى وصفت أقول انّا نغذو
المريض الذى هذه حاله منذ أوّل المرض بكشك الشعير بعد أن نحذر ونعلم
بالحدود التى علّمناها بقراط هل يحتاج ذلك المريض إلى أن يكون مع ماء كشك
الشعير ثفله أو يكفيه الماء فقط فإنّ بقراط يذمّ فى هذا الباب قوما من الأطبّاء ٦
كانوا يجفّفون أوّلا أبدان المرضى فى الأيّام الأول من المرض كما قد يفعل ذلك
كثيرا أهل دهرنا من الأطبّاء ثمّ يغذونهم بغذاء ذى قدر بالقرب من وقت المنتهى
ولا فرق فى هذا الكلام بين قولى منتهى وبين قولى بحران فإنّ بقراط قد بيّن أنّ ٧
الذى ينبغى أن يفعل ضدّ ما كان يفعل أولآئك أعنى أن ينقص من الغذاء إذا قرب
وقت المنتهى حتّى أنّا كثيرا ما لا نغذو المريض بتّة فى يوم بحران فقد قال
بقراط فى هذا الباب قولا أنّا واصفه بلفظه وهو هذا إنّ من أعظم جميع ما أفيدكه
عندى نفعا أنّه لا ينبغى أن تمنع المريض فى الأيّام الأول من مرضه ثمّ
من بعد الأحساء على أنّها تختلف وأنت مزمع بعد قليل أن تغذوه ببعض تلك
الأحساء ولم يطلق القول فيقول انّه لا ينبغى أن يمنع المريض فى أوّل مرضه من ٨
الأحساء لكن استثنى فقال وأنت مزمع بعد قليل أن تغذوه بالأحساء يعنى بذلك
المريض الذى تضطرّ إلى أن تغذوه من قبل وقت منتهى مرضه فإنّ المريض الذى ٩
يحتمل أن يبقى من غير أن تغذوه ليس ينبغى أن تقتصر على أن تمنعه من الحسو فى
الأيّام الثلاثة من مرضه دون أن تمنعه منه فى اليوم الرابع أيضا إذا كنت تتوقّع له

1 يترك] يقول B : corr. B¹ — 2 إلى استعماله] ان يستعمل B — 5 منذ] من B
نحذر] نحدد A — 6 ابقراط B — 7 يكتفيه A — 9 كثيرا] اكثر B — 12 لا om. B
13 post هذا^II add. ابقراط B — 14 ثمّ om. B — 15 بعد^I] بعض B — على] وعلى A
18 الذى^II om. B — 19 ليس] بيسير B — 20 له om. B

must be left until it settles down. Similarly, when the patient is in need of bleeding or of a purge, he is not fed until the requisite remedy has been applied.

Suppose, however, that we have a patient whose disease is expected 5
to reach its crisis on the ninth, eleventh or fourteenth day, and who is not in need of any of those treatments that I mentioned. I say that whoever is in this state is fed on barley gruel from the start of his illness, after we have taken the precaution of determining by the rules taught us by Hippocrates whether he requires barley groats together with his barley water, or whether the barley water by itself is enough for him.

On this point Hippocrates blames a number of doctors who used 6
to start by desiccating the bodies of their patients in the early stages of their illness[1] – a thing which is often done by our medical contemporaries – and who then give them sizeable quantities of food when the climax is near. – There is, incidentally, no difference in this account of mine between my use of the terms *muntahā* – climax – and *buḥrān* – crisis.

Hippocrates has made it clear that the proper treatment is, in fact, 7
the opposite to that used by these doctors – I mean that, at the approach of the climax, the patient should be given less food and on the day of the crisis he is often not to be fed at all. On this point he made a remark which I will quote word for word. It runs as follows: "One of the most useful of all the pieces of advice that I can give you is that you should not deny your patient the various forms of broth from the initial stage of his disease onwards when you are planning soon afterwards to feed him on some of those same types of broth."[2]
He does not make the statement absolute and claim that the patient 8
should not be denied broth in the initial stage of his illness. Rather, he adds a qualification and says: "when you are planning soon afterwards to feed him on broth", the reference being to the man who has to be fed before the climax of his illness. But those who are capable 9
of remaining without food should be kept off broth not just on the first three days of the illness but on the fourth as well, when the crisis

[1] Cf. De diaet. in morb. acut., I 122, 2 Kw.

[2] τοῦτο οὖν ἡγεῦμαι μέγιστον διδακτήριον, ὅτι οὐ στερητέαι αἱ πρῶται ἡμέραι τοῦ ῥυφήματος ἢ τοίου ἢ τοίου τοῖσι μέλλουσιν ὀλίγον ὕστερον ῥυφήμασιν ἢ σιτίοισι χρῆσθαι. De diaet. in morb. acut., I 128, 19–129, 2 Kw.

البحران فى اليوم الخامس وعلى هذا المثال قد يمنع المريض من الحسو فى اليوم
الخامس أيضا وفى اليوم السادس وفى اليوم السابع كثيرا إذا كان قويّا وكان يتوقّع له
البحران فى تلك الأيّام ويصرّح بالذمّ واللوم لمن يبتدئ بتغذية المريض فى أحد ١٠
هذه الأيّام بكشك الشعير بعد أن قد سبق فجفّف بدنه بالمنع من الغذاء
واستعماله لهذا اللفظ أعنى قوله سبق فجفّف بدنه جارٍ على حقيقة ما يدلّ عليه
هذا اللفظ وذلك أنّهم إذا كانوا يضطرّون إلى أن يغذوا المريض فى الوقت الذى ١١
كان ينبغى أن يمنعوه فيه من الغذاء لقرب وقت منتهى مرضه فبيّن أنّهم قد
كانوا سبقوا فجفّفوا بدنه وذلك أنّه إن كان يحتمل أن يبقى من غير غذاء فليس
يحتاج إلى التغذية وإن كان يحتاج وبالواجب يغذونه فبيّن أنّهم قد جفّفوا بدنه
فى الأيّام الأول من مرضه وذلك أنّهم لا يقدرون أن يقولوا انّ القياس يدلّ على ١٢
أنّه ينبغى أن يغذو نحو وقت منتهى المرض من يحتمل أن يبقى إلى أن يأتيه البحران من
غير غذاء فالذى يغذو المريض إذًا على أنّه لا يحتمل أن يبقى مخطئ فى قتله إيّاه
بالجوع فى أوّل مرضه والذى يغذوه بقراط إذًا منذ أوّل مرضه إنّما هو من ١٣
لا يطمع أن يبقى له قوّته إلى أن يأتيه البحران من غير أن يرزأ من الغذاء شيئا
البتّة وهذا هو المعنى الذى يشير إليه بقراط بقوله خلاء العروق فى ذلك الكتاب
كلّه أعنى كتابه فى الأمراض الحادّة

٣ فقد تبيّن إذًا أنّ الرجل الذى ظنّ بابقراط أنّه كان يغذو المريض فى كلّ يوم قد بلغ من جهله أنّه لا يعرف معانى الألفاظ وينبغى لك أن تعلّمه أنّ ما يعنى بقراط فى قوله يسبق فيستعمل خلاء العروق إنّما هو أن يسبق فيستعمل ترك الغذاء فإنّك إن علمت ذلك فهمت قول بقراط وهو هذا فإنّى أقول انّ ابتداء بتناول المريض للحسو منذ أوّل الأمر أجود من أن يسبق فيستعمل خلاء العروق ثمّ يبتدئ بتناول الحسو فى اليوم الثالث من مرضه أو فى الرابع أو فى الخامس أو فى السادس أو فى السابع إلّا أن يتقدّم بحران المرض فيكون فى هذه المدّة فإنّه

2 له *om.* B 4 قد *om.* B فجفّف] وجفف B من] عن B 5 جارٍ] جارى A : جاريا B : *correxi* 7 يكون B منتهى وقت *trsp.* B 8 إن *om.* A 12 إذاً *om.* B لا *om.* B *post* مخطئ *add.* مسمى B : *del.* B', *ut vid.* : مسىء *legerit* Strohmaier 13 فالذى B 15 البتّة] بتة B 18 فينبغى B 19 ما يعنى] معنى B 20 علمت] عملت A : علمته B : *correxi* فهم B *post* هذا *add.* بقراط B

is expected on the fifth day. In the same way patients are denied broth on the fifth day also and on the sixth and often on the seventh, when they are strong and the crisis is expected during that period.

Hippocrates plainly reproves and blames those who begin to feed 10
their patients on barley gruel on one of those days, after previously
having desiccated their bodies by keeping them from food. His use
of this expression, I mean the phrase, "having previously desiccated
the body"[1], accords with the exact significance of the terms. Those 11
doctors have been forced to feed the patient at a time when, because
of the proximity of the climax of his disease, he should have been
prevented from eating and so it is clear that earlier they desiccated his
body. For if he was capable of remaining without food, then he did
not need to be fed. But if he did need food and had to be fed, obviously
they must have desiccated his body in the early stages of the disease.
For they cannot claim it to be shown by reason that towards the 12
climax of the illness one should feed a patient who is capable of
remaining without food until the crisis arrives. So then the doctor who
feeds his patient on the grounds that he is unable to survive (without
food) has done wrong in starving him to death at the beginning of his
illness. Those whom Hippocrates feeds from the start are the ones 13
whose strength is not expected to last until the crisis if they are given
no food at all. This, incidentally, is what he means by his expression,
"emptying of the veins"[2], throughout all that book, I mean his work
"On Acute Diseases".

3. It is obvious, then, that the man who thinks that Hippocrates used to feed his patients every day is so far sunk in ignorance as not to know what the words mean. You must teach him that, when Hippocrates says, "he first empties the veins", he means that he starts by using starvation treatment. When you grasp that, you can understand what he means in the following sentence: "I say that for the patient to start by taking broth from the beginning is better than for him first to be made to fast and then to begin to take broth on the third, fourth, fifth, sixth or seventh day of his illness, unless the crisis has

[1] προταριχεύσαντες De diaet. in morb. acut., I 122, 4 Kw.

[2] κενεαγγίη De diaet. in morb. acut., I 114, 15 Kw. al.

إن تقدّم كون البحران فبيّن أنّ ابتداء بتناول الحسو فى أحد هذه الأيّام صواب
أمّا أنا فأرى وبالله أقسم أنّ بقراط قد استعمل فى هذا الكلام من الإيضاح ٢
والبيان ما لا يخفى معه على صبىّ فضلا عمّن سواه أنّه يدلّ أنّ تغيّر التدبير إنّما
يضرّ بمن امتنع من الغذاء فى الأيّام الأول من مرضه إن لم يتقدّم فيأتيه البحران
قبل أن يغيّر تدبيره أعنى لم ينحطّ مرضه وينتقص بوجه من الوجوه وذلك أنّ
المرض إن كان قد انحطّ ونقص فاستعمال كشك الشعير صواب وإن كان المريض قد
منع من الغذاء سبعة أيّام فضلا عن أن يكون إنّما منع ثلاثة أيّام أو أربعة فقد ٣
تبيّن أنّ بقراط قد يمنع كثيرا من المرضى من الغذاء بتّة لا فى الأيّام الثلاثة الأول
من مرضهم فقط لكن إلى اليوم السابع إذا كان يتوقّع مجىء البحران قبل سقوط
القوّة وهذا هو الباب الذى يذمّ فيه أرسسطراطس دكسفس وافلونس ٤
تلميذى بقراط وأشياعهما ويذمّ أيضا معهم قوما آخرين من الأطبّاء أعنى أنّهم
يقتلون المريض بالجوع إلّا أن ترى أنّ منع المريض من الغذاء سبعة أيّام منذ أوّل
مرضه تجويع يسير أمّا أنا فأرى أنّ تجويع المريض خمسة أيّام كبير إلّا أنّا قد نجد ٥
بقراط لا يذمّ من يبتدئ بتغذية المريض فى اليوم السابع بعد أن يكون البحران قد
تقدّم فكان وأمّا هذا الطبيب العجيب الذى يرى فى نفسه أنّه أعلم بطريق
تدبير بقراط للأمراض الحادّة من أرسسطراطس ومن تلامذة بقراط يرى أنّ
بقراط يغذو جميع المرضى فى كلّ يوم وبقراط يصيح أن يخطئ من يبتدئ بتغذية
المريض بالحسو فى اليوم السابع إذا كان قد تقدّم فكان البحران وأنا واضع شيئا من ٦
كلامه فى ذلك فأثبت فى ذهنك وتدبّره قال بقراط ثمّ من بعد إن كان يجد المريض

1 كون] فكان B تناوله للحسو B 3 التبيين B 4 إن] من AB
5 لم] لن A 6 تنقص B 7 إنّما *om.* B 10 يذمّ] تقدم A دكسفس]
وكسنقر B 11 اشياعهم A قوم A 12 ترى أنّ *om.* B 13 كبير]
كثير B قد *om.* A 16 الحادّة *om.* B يرى] *fort.* فيرى *scribendum est*
17 يصيح] يصرّح *correxerit* Strohmaier أن] لن B: *fort.* ان لن *scribendum est*
19 فى II] فيه B قال *om.* B

already passed during this period"[1]. If it has, then obviously it is right to begin to take broth on one of those days.

My opinion – and I swear to it by God[2] – is that Hippocrates 2
has made this account of his so clear and obvious that not even a child, much less anyone else, should find it obscure. He is showing that a change in treatment can only harm a patient who has been kept from food at the beginning of his illness, unless before the change is made the crisis has already passed, that is to say the disease has diminished and abated in some way or other. For in that case it is right to use barley gruel, even if the patient has been kept from food for seven days, let alone when he has only been kept from it for three or four
days. It is obvious, then, that Hippocrates denies many of his 3
patients all food, not merely in the first three days of their illness but until the seventh day, in cases where the arrival of the crisis is expected to precede the collapse of their strength.

This is the point on which Erasistratus blames Dexippus and 4
Apollonius, pupils of Hippocrates, their followers and other doctors as well. He accuses them of killing their patients by starvation[3] – unless you think that to keep a sick man from eating for
seven days from the beginning of his illness is a small fast. For my part, 5
I think it serious enough to make him fast for five days, but we find that Hippocrates does not blame those who begin to feed their patients on the seventh day, after the crisis is past. But this admirable physician, who thinks to himself that he knows more about Hippocrates' treatment of acute diseases than Erasistratus and Hippocrates' pupils, holds that Hippocrates feeds every one of his patients every day. Hippocrates, however, cries out that it is a mistake to begin to feed a patient with broth on the seventh day, unless[4] the crisis is past.

I shall quote a remark of his on that point, which you should keep 6
well in mind and think over. He says: "Afterwards, if the patient

---

[1] *φημὶ γὰρ ἄμεινον εἶναι αὐτίκα ἄρξασθαι ῥυφεῖν τὸ ἐπίπαν μᾶλλον ἢ προκενεαγγήσαντα ἄρξασθαι τοῦ ῥυφήματος τριταῖον ἢ τεταρταῖον ἢ πεμπταῖον ἢ ἑκταῖον ἢ ἑβδομαῖον, ἤν γε μὴ προκριθῇ ἡ νοῦσος ἐν τούτῳ τῷ χρόνῳ.* De diaet. in morb. acut., I 121, 16–20 Kw.

[2] *νὴ Δία* (?).

[3] *τὰ γὰρ εἰς Ἀπολλώνιον καὶ Δέξιππον τοὺς Ἱπποκράτους μαθητὰς εἰρημένα κατὰ τὸ πρῶτον Περὶ πυρετῶν Ἐρασιστράτῳ τὴν διαβολὴν τῆς λιμαγχονίας εἰς Ἱπποκράτην τὸν διδάσκαλον ἀναφερομένην ἔχει.* CMG V 9, 1 p. 145, 22–24.

[4] The text gives 'if'; a negative is suggested in the Apparatus.

وجعا أو ظهر فيه شيء من الأعراض المخوّفة فينبغي أن يعطى الحسو وهو ليس
بالغليظ ولا بالكثير من بعد اليوم السابع إن كان قويّا وهذا الكلام يوجد فى ٧
النسخ مختلفا لأنّه يوجد فى بعضها فيه زيادة حرف زائد فيما بين قوله ولا بالكثير
وبين قوله من بعد اليوم السابع وذلك حتّى يكون نسق الكلام على هذا المثال
وذلك من بعد اليوم السابع إن كان قويّا ويوجد فى بعض النسخ وليس معه ذلك
الحرف على المثال الأوّل الذى وضعناه عليه والمعنى المفهوم من هاتين النسختين
جميعا معنى واحد وهو أنّ بقراط أمر أن يكون إعطاؤنا ماء كشك الشعير لمن كان ٨
مرضه ذا خطر أو كان يجد وجعا من بعد اليوم السابع لا قبله إذا كانت قوّته قويّة
تحتمل الإمساك عن الغذاء هذه المدّة فقد تبيّن فى هذا الموضع أيضا أنّ بقراط قد ٩
جعل ابتداء تغذيته لبعض المرضى بماء كشك الشعير من بعد اليوم السابع ويقتصر
به قبل ذلك إمّا على ماء العسل وإمّا على سكنجبين وإمّا على الماء القراح على
نحو ما يرى الحاجة تدعو إلى كلّ واحد من هذه الأشربة فقد يصف بقراط من
بعد هذا الكلام الأغراض التى ينبغي أن نقصد إليها فى استعمال هذه الأشربة
٤ فالأجود إذاً كان أن تسألنى ما بال بقراط يستعمل فى أصحاب الأمراض
الحادّة هذا التدبير اللطيف كلّه لا كما سألتنى ما بال بقراط يغذو أصحاب
الأمراض الحادّة فى كلّ يوم إذ كان لا يغذو صاحب المرض الحادّ فى كلّ يوم
إلّا فى الندرة وإذا غذاه أيضا فى كلّ يوم كان تدبيره له أيضا تدبيرا لطيفا وتقدر ٢
أن تعرف حقيقة ذلك إذا أنت تدبّرت كلاما قاله أنا واضعه لك بلفظه قال بقراط
يكتفى أن يعطى المريض فى أوّل مرضه مقدارا ليس بالكثير ولا بالغليظ لكن كيما
يكون قد ورد البدن شيء بسبب العادة ولا يفرط فيه خلاء العروق فهذا الكلام منه ٣
يدلّ على أنّه إذا أعطى صاحب المرض الحادّ من ماء كشك الشعير شيئا ليس
بالكثير ولا بالغليظ فإنّما يفعل ذلك كيما لا يفرط عليه خلاء العروق يعنى الحمية

6 وضعناه] وصفناه A   8 إذا] اذ B   8 sq. قد . . . قويّة *om.* B   10 جعل] يجعل B
11 سكنجبين] السكنجبين B   على[IV] *om.* B   13 بعد *om.* B   14 إذاً كان *trsp.* B
15 بال بقراط] باله B   18 إذا] ان B   واضعه] واصفه A   بقراط قال *trsp.* B   20 فيه] فى A   22 وانما A

experiences pain, or if there appears some alarming complication, he
should be given broth, though this should not be thick or in any large
amount, after the seventh day, if he is strong"[1]. This sentence is found 7
differently worded in the manuscripts[2]. In some an additional phrase
is inserted between the words, "or in any large amount", and, "after the
seventh day", so that it runs: "and that can be done after the seventh
day, if the patient is strong". Other manuscripts do not include this
extra phrase and give the sentence in the original form that we quoted.
But the meaning to be understood from both these versions is one and
the same. Hippocrates is recommending us to give barley water to 8
those who are suffering from serious diseases or who are experiencing
pain, after the seventh day and not before it, when their strength is
sufficient to support a fast for this period.

Another point that is plain here is that Hippocrates starts feeding 9
some of his patients after the seventh day on barley water, when
before he has confined the diet to honey water, oxymel or pure water,
as he thinks the need demands.

He next describes what our object should be in the employment of these drinks[3].

4. It would be better, then, for you to ask me why Hippocrates
uses all this light regimen in the case of those who are suffering from
acute diseases, than to ask, as you have, why he feeds such patients
every day. For in fact it is only rarely that he does this, and even then
the regimen is still light. You will be in a position to recognise the truth 2
of that when you have studied a sentence of his which I propose to
quote for you verbatim. Hippocrates said: "It is enough that at the
beginning of his illness the patient should be given no great quantity
of food, nor should this be thick. He should, however, be given something
so that his body may receive some nourishment for habit's sake
and the emptying of the veins not be carried too far."[4] This remark 3
of his shows that when he gives those who suffer from acute diseases
a small quantity of barley gruel, which must not be thick, he does so

---

[1] ἔπειτα, ἢν μὲν ἄλγημα ἐνῇ ἢ τῶν ἐπικινδύνων τι ἐμφαίνηται, διδόναι τὸ ῥύφημα μήτε παχὺ μήτε πολύ, μετὰ δὲ τὴν ἑβδόμην, ἢν ἰσχύῃ. De diaet. in morb. acut., I 118, 14–17 Kw.

[2] For Galen's concern with variant readings in this text v. CMG V 9, 1 p. 119, 4sqq. 182, 25sqq. 189, 14sqq. 205, 29sqq.

[3] De diaet. in morb. acut., I 134, 7sq. Kw.

[4] πλῆθος δὲ ἀρκεῖ κατ' ἀρχὰς διδόναι μὴ πολὺ μηδὲ ὑπέρπαχυ, ἀλλ' ὅσον εἵνεκα τοῦ ἔθεος ἐσιέναι τι καὶ κενεαγγίην μὴ γενέσθαι πολλήν. De diaet. in morb. acut., I 114, 13–16 Kw.

والإمساك عن الطعام فالأمر عنده أنّ المريض إذا تدبّر بهذا التدبير أيضا فهو على ٤
سبيل من الحمية والإقلال من الطعم والتدبير اللطيف إلّا أنّ ذلك ليس بالكثير
المفرط كما لو لم ينل من ماء كشك الشعير ولا هذا المقدار اليسير فأخطر ببالك مريضا ٥
من المرضى الذين حالهم فى مرضهم الحال التى يأتى معها البحران فى اليوم الرابع
عشر وأنّ ذلك المريض إنّما يعطى سكرجة صغيرة فى اليوم من ماء كشك
الشعير على طريق الشراب لا على طريق الطعام وذلك أيضا ليس فى كلّ يوم
وذلك أنّه لا يسقى فى اليوم الأوّل من مرضه شيئا منه دون أن ينحدر الطعام الأوّل إن
كان فى معدته طعام أو يفصد إن كان محتاجا إلى الفصد أو يسكن وجع إن كان
به ولا يسقاه أيضا فى الأيّام التى يمنع فيها من إسقائه إيّاه عظم نوبة الحمّى على ٦
أنّه لو كان يسقى فى كلّ يوم من تلك الأربعة عشر يوما تلك السكرجة الصغيرة
من ماء كشك الشعير لقد كان ذلك المقدار على الحال الذى يسقـــاه فى تلك الأيّام
كلّها أقلّ من مقدار هذا الغذاء الذى يغذو به أكثر أهل زماننا هذا من الأطبّاء
كثيرا من أصحاب الأمراض الحادّة فى يوم واحد وذلك أنّا نجدهم كثيرا يحسون ٧
المريض أوّلا قدحا مملوءا من الحنطة التى يقال لها خندروس وقد هرست وطبخت
وطيّبت بماء العسل ثمّ يحسونه من بعد ذلك من تلك الحنطة حسوا آخر يسمّونه
الطحين ثمّ يطعمونه خصى الديوك وأجنحتها وفراخ الحمام والشفانين وأترك أن
أذكر الآن ما يطعمونه فى خلال هذا من بصلتين أو ثلاث من البصل الذى يقال له بصل
الزيز ومن السمك الذى يطعمونه كثيرا من أجناس السمك الذى يقال له الرعّاد
ولسان الثور والابرسيون وسائر أنواع السمك فأكله واحدة من هذه الأكلات التى ٨
يطعمونها المرضى أصحاب هذا التدبير أكثر وأقوى من ماء كشك الشعير الذى يسقاه

1 الطعم B   2 من الطعم *om.* B   4 الحال التى *om.* B   5 *ante* اليوم *add.* كل B   6 أيضا *om.* B   8 و [أو^{II} B   11 حال B   سقى [يسقاه B   14 خندرس B   16 والشفانين وفراخ الحمام *trsp.* B   انزل [أترك B: *corr.* B'   19 الابرسيون] *fort.* الابرسون (πράσον) *legendum est*   فأكلة *legerit* Strohmaier   20 يطعمها الان [يطعمونها B

simply to stop the emptying of the veins, that is the process of prohi-
bitive and restrictive diet, from being carried to excess. His view is 4
that even when the patient is under this regimen, he is still in the way
of being subject to prohibitive diet, food restriction and light treat-
ment, though this is not taken to excessive lengths as it would be if
he were not provided with even this small quantity of gruel.

Now imagine to yourself a certain patient who is one of those whose 5
condition is such that the crisis of their disease will occur on the four-
teenth day. This man is only given a small saucer of barley water
during the day, by way of liquid and not by way of food. Nor does he
get this saucer every day. For he is not given anything to drink on the
first day of his illness until what food, if any, he already has in his
stomach subsides, or until he is bled, if he needs this, or until any pain
that he may be experiencing is alleviated[1]. Nor does he get this
to drink on the days when this is prevented by the violence of his fits
of fever. But even if he were given that small saucer of barley water 6
to drink on each of the fourteen days of his illness, yet even so the
quantity of what was given him throughout the whole of that period
would be less than that of the food which the majority of our contem-
porary doctors provide many of those suffering from acute diseases on
a single day. For we find them often starting by giving the patient a 7
bowl filled with what is known as *χόνδρος* wheat, that has been
brayed, cooked and flavoured with honey water. Next he is given an-
other form of broth made from that wheat and called *al-ṭaḥīn*, then
cocks' testicles and wings, together with young pigeons and doves[2].
I will not mention the two or three so-called *zīz* onions[3], with which
he is provided in the intervals, together with the various kinds of
torpedo fish which are often supplied[4], together with bugloss and
leeks[5], as well as the other kinds of fish. A single one of the dishes given 8
by these dieticians to their patients provides more and stronger

[1] *οὓς δ' ἤτοι κενῶσαι διὰ φλεβοτομίας ἢ γαστρὸς ἀναγκαῖόν ἐστιν ἢ ὀδυνωμένους παῦσαι, τούτοις μὴ πρότερον διδόναι πτισάνην* CMG V 9, 1 p. 140, 21–23.

[2] *καθάπερ οὐδ' ἄλλῳ τινὶ τῶν εἰθισμένων δίδοσθαι τοῖς ἀρρώστοις ὑπὸ τῶν νῦν ἰατρῶν, οἷον ᾠῶν καὶ ὄρχεων ἀλεκτρυόνων καὶ πτερῶν ἰχθύων τε καὶ περιστερῶν νεογνῶν, ὅσα τ' ἄλλα τοιαῦτα.* CMG V 9, 1 p. 146, 27–29.

[3] *σκίλλα* v. XII 125, 4–8 K.

[4] The text or the translation may be at fault here, in that the construction of the phrase suggests that what follows should be a list of fish.

[5] Reading الابرسون (*πράσον*).

المريض فى مدّة مرضه كلّها الذى قد تقدّم بقراط فيه أن يكون يسيرا رقيقا لا
غليظا كثيرا ويتقدّم أيضا مع ذلك أن لا يسقى المريض ذلك فى جميع الأيّام كما
قد بيّنّا

٥ وإذا كان بقراط قد يبلغ من تلطيفه للغذاء منذ أوّل المرض هذا المبلغ
كلّه حتّى يكون ما ينيله المريض إنّما هو بقدر ما يكون قد ورد البدن شىء بسبب
العادة ولا يفرط الخوى عليه فكم بالحرىّ يكون تلطيفه لتدبيره إذا مرّت الأيّام فقد ٢
قال بقراط انّ من كان منتهى مرضه يأتى بدءا فينبغى أن يدبّر بالتدبير اللطيف
بدءا ومن كان منتهى مرضه يتأخّر فينبغى أن يمنع من الغذاء فى وقت المنتهى وقبله
بقليل ويدبّر قبل ذلك تدبيرا أغلظ كيما يبقى فإذا كان فى الوقت الذى يحتاج فيه ٣
إلى التدبير الذى هو أغلظ إنّما يسقى من ماء كشك الشعير مقدارا يسيرا جدّا حتّى
يكون التدبير قريبا من تدبير من يمنع الغذاء بتّة ثمّ كان ينقص من هذا المقدار أيضا
دائما إلى أن يبلغ إلى وقت المنتهى ثمّ يأمر بالامتناع فى وقت المنتهى من الغذاء فقد ٤
تبيّن لك أنّ مبلغ تدبيره فى اللطافة مبلغ عظيم جدّا فقول ارسسطراطس على
هذا القياس أشبه بالحقّ وهو ما قاله من أنّ آل بقراط يتوقّون كلّ غذاء لأنّهم
كانوا يرون أنّ الغذاء إنّما هو بمنزلة الوقيد للحمّ ولذلك لم يكونوا يكادون يغذون ٥
أصحاب الأمراض الحادّة إلى أن يجوز اليوم السابع فإن خافوا على قوّته أن
تخور اقتصروا به على ماء العسل ولم يكونوا يغذون المريض الذى تكون مدّة مرضه
إلى السابع كما قلت بماء كشك الشعير إلّا فى الندرة وأمّا الأمراض التى يكون ٦
انقضاؤها فى أربعة عشر يوما فليس يمكن أن يقتصر بالمريض فيها على
التغذية بماء العسل لكنّهم كانوا يقتصرون بالمريض الذى هذه حاله على كشك
الشعير فيغذونه به من أوّل مرضه ولا يقرّبونه شيئا غيره من الأغذية
بتّة وليس البحث عن هذا التدبير هل بقراط فيه مصيب أو مخطئ من كلامى ٧

1 يتقدم A   سيرا [يسيرا B   4 فاذ [وإذا B   7 *ante* من *add.* كل B
يأتى *om.* B   9 بتدبير [تدبيرا B   فان [فإذا B   11 منه [بتّة B
12 بالامتناع *post* المنتهى II *trsp.* B   13 اراسسطراطس B   14 *ante* يتوقّون
add. كانوا B   15 أنّ *om.* B   للحمى [للحم B

nourishment than the barley gruel that Hippocrates' patient drinks
during the whole course of his illness and which, on his recommenda-
tion, should be small in quantity and thin, not thick and abundant.
He also recommends that the patient should not be given the gruel to
drink every day, as we have shown.

5. Hippocrates, then, has developed the principle of refinement
in diet from the start of the disease so far that what the patient
receives is only enough to let his body have something for habit's
sake and to prevent it from becoming too empty. How much more,
then, does he refine this diet as the days pass. For he has said that 2
where the climax comes early the patient should from the start be
treated with a light diet and where it is postponed he should be kept
from food at the time of the climax and a little before it[1]. Earlier he
should be treated with a more solid diet, in order to keep him alive.
But at the time when he needs this latter type of treatment he is only 3
given a very small portion indeed of barley water to drink, in order
that his regimen may approximate to that of the man who is kept off
food altogether. Then even this portion would be constantly diminished
until the climax is reached, at which stage Hippocrates tells us to
forbid him food.

It must be clear to you, then, that Hippocrates' regimen is very 4
light indeed and, following this line of argument, Erasistratus'
dictum comes close to the truth. For he said that the followers of
Hippocrates were wary of all kinds of food, since they thought that
the position of food was like that of fuel in relation to heat. Conse- 5
quently they scarcely fed at all those who were suffering from an acute
disease until after the seventh day, though if it was feared that the
patient's strength might sink, they kept him on honey water. Only on
rare occasions, as I said, did they give barley water to someone
suffering from a seven day disease. But in the case of an illness which 6
lasts for fourteen days it is impossible to keep the patient on a diet of
honey water. Rather, they used to confine a man in this condition to
barley gruel, which he was given from the start of his illness and he
was given no other kind of food at all.

To enquire whether Hippocrates was right or wrong in pre- 7
scribing this regimen is not relevant to my present discussion. For

[1] Aphor. I 10 *ὁκόσοισι μὲν οὖν αὐτίκα ἡ ἀκμὴ, αὐτίκα λεπτῶς διαιτῆν. ὁκόσοισι δὲ ἐς ὕστερον ἡ ἀκμὴ, ἐς ἐκεῖνο, καὶ πρὸ ἐκείνου σμικρὸν, ἀφαιρετέον·* (IV 464, 7–9 L.).

هذا فى شىء فأمّا الأمر الذى قصدت له فقد وضح وتبيّن وهو أنّ بقراط أشدّ
استعمالا من جميع من عزّ قبله من الأطبّاء للتدبير اللطيف وأنّ ارسسطراطس لم
يكذب عليه وعلى آله

٦ وتقدر أن تعلم أيضا أنّه كان يغذو بعض المرضى بماء كشك الشعير ومعه ثفله
ويغذو بعضهم بمائه فقط ويحمى بعضهم من ماء الشعير أيضا من كلام ذكره فى
كتابه فى تدبير الأمراض الحادّة فإنّه قال أوّلا هذا القول وطريق الرفد فى أكثر
الأمر طريق واحد لمن يستعمل ماء الشعير ومعه ثفله ولمن يستعمل ماءه فقط ولمن لا
يستعمل واحدا منهما بتّة لكن يقتصر على ما يشرب وربّما كان طريق
الرفد مختلفا ثمّ قال بعد فى صفته ماء العسل هذا القول وإن تجنّبت الاحساء ٢
واقتصرت على ماء العسل فى هذه الأمراض كان صوابك كثيرا وخطاؤك قليلا غير
كثير ثمّ قال بعد هذا القول فى صفتـه للسكنجبين فأمّا من يقتصر على التدبير ٣
بما يشرب فقـط من غير أن يرزأ شيئا من الأحسـاء فلهذا السبب لا يوافقه أنّ
يقتصر على ذلك دائما ثمّ قال بعد هذا فى صفته للحمّام هذا القول انّ استعمال ٤
الاستحمام فى الحمّام لمن يستعمل ماء الشعير مع ثفله أمكن منه لمن يقتصر على
مائه وقد يقدر من يقتصر على ماء الشعير كثيرا على استعمال الحمّام فأمّا من
يقتصر على ما يشرب فقط فلا يكاد يقدر على استعمال الحمّام فنراك تحتاج ٥
مع هذا الكلام إلى أن أجيبك بكلام غيره من ذلك الكتاب أعنى كتاب تدبير
الأمراض الحادّة أو من غيره من كتبه يتقدّم بقراط أن يقتصر بكثير من المرضى فى

2 عزّ قبله] عرفنا B post استعمالا *add.* للامرين جميعا B : جميعا *del.* B'
5 كلام *om.* B 6 post القول *add.* بقراط B 9 post الرفد *add.* طريقا A لماء B
10 وفى] و B ante كان *add.* فان B قليلا *om.* B 13 على *om.* B
بعد هذا *om.* B 16 فنراك] اتراك *ut vid.* B 18 وأن] و B بكثير *om.* B

the point that I wanted to make has been clearly demonstrated. It is that Hippocrates made more use of light regimen than did any famous doctor before him, nor did Erasistratus lie in what he said about him and his school.

6. You can also learn that Hippocrates used to feed some of his
patients on barley water together with barley groats and some on
barley water alone, while others he prevented even from drinking this.
This is to be found in the account in his book "On Regimen in Acute
Diseases". First of all he writes: "The adjutory methods, for the most
part, are the same for those who employ barley water together with
barley groats, for those who use barley water alone and for those who
make no use either of the one or the other at all, but confine their
patients to drinking (water). Sometimes, though, these methods do
vary."[1] Afterwards in an account of honey water he makes the 2
following remark: "If you avoid broth and restrict yourself to honey
water in these diseases you will be in the right for the most part and
what mistakes you do make will be scant and few."[2] Then in his 3
account of oxymel he writes: "For this reason it is not always suitable
to restrict the diet of the patient to drink alone without giving him
any broth."[3] Next, in his description of baths he writes: "To bathe 4
in the baths is more proper for those who use barley water together
with barley groats than for those who confine themselves to barley
water, and, though these latter can, in fact, often use the baths, this
can scarcely be done by those who confine themselves to drinking
(water)."[4]

I see, however, that in addition to this account you require my 5
reply to include other statements taken from that book, I mean the
work "On Regimen in Acute Diseases", or from others of Hippocrates' works. Hippocrates recommends that many patients should

---

[1] *μάλα μὲν οὖν τὰ πλεῖστα παραπλήσιοί εἰσιν αἱ τιμωρίαι τοῖσί τε οὔλῃσι πτισάνῃσι χρεωμένοισι τοῖσί τε χυλῷ αὐτῷ· τοῖσι δὲ μηδετέρῳ τούτων, ἀλλὰ ποτῷ μοῦνον, ἔστιν ὅπῃ καὶ διαφερόντως τιμωρητέον.* De diaet. in morb. acut., I 118, 3–6 Kw.

[2] *ἄνευ μὲν ῥυφημάτων μελικρήτῳ χρεώμενος ἀντ' ἄλλου ποτοῦ ἐν ταύτῃσι τῇσι νούσοισι πολλὰ ἂν εὐτυχοίης καὶ οὐκ ἂν πολλὰ ἀτυχοίης.* De diaet. in morb. acut., I 137, 3–5 Kw.

[3] *τοῖσι δὲ ποτῷ μοῦνον διαιτωμένοισιν ἄνευ ῥυφημάτων διὰ τόδε οὐκ ἐπιτήδειόν ἐστιν αἰεὶ μοῦνον χρῆσθαι τούτῳ·* De diaet. in morb. acut., I 140, 6–8 Kw.

[4] *χρῆσθαι δὲ λουτροῖσι τοῖσι οὔλῃσι πτισάνῃσι χρεωμένοισι παρὰ πολὺ μᾶλλον ἐνδέχεται ἢ τοῖσι χυλῷ μοῦνον χρεωμένοισιν· ἐνδέχεται δὲ καὶ τούτοισιν ἐνίοτε· ἥκιστα δὲ τοῖσι ποτῷ μοῦνον χρεωμένοις·* De diaet. in morb. acut., I 144, 21–145, 2 Kw.

مدّة مرضهم كلّها على ما يشرب فقط من غير أن يرزؤوا شيئا من الطعام بتّة
أمّا أنا فيمكنني أن أجمع من كلامه فى ذلك ما يجىء منه كتاب تامّ لكنّى أعلم
أنّى إن فعلت ذلك أبرمتك فأنا راجع إلى ما كنت قصدت إليه فأجتهد فيما قصدت
له فأجتهد أن أختصر منه تدبير بقراط للأمراض الحادّة كلّه فى جمل مقتصدة
قليل عددها فأقول إنّ بقراط يرى أنّ من أعظم الناس خطاء من حمل المريض ٦
فى أوّل مرضه على أن يمتنع من الغذاء ثلاثة أيّام أو أربعة ثمّ يغذوه من بعد
ذلك وقد قرب وقت منتهى مرضه وذلك أنّه إنّما ينبغى إمّا أن لا يمنع المريض من
الغذاء إن كانت قوّته لا تفى بمقاومة المرض أو إن كانت تفى بذلك فأن يمنع من
الغذاء على ما دبّر فيه منذ أوّل المرض إلى أن ينضج مرضه إن كان ذلك يكون فى
اليوم الخامس أو فى السادس أو فى السابع فهذا هو رأى بقراط وأمّا رأى غيره من ٧
الأطبّاء فتعرفه ممّا وصفه بقراط وذلك أنّه قال فى كتابه فى تدبير الأمراض
الحادّة هذا القول وقد أعرف كثيرا من الأطبّاء يفعل ضدّ ما ينبغى أن يفعل
وذلك أنّهم كلّهم يجفّفون أبدان المرضى منذ أوّل المرض يومين أو ثلاثة أو أكثر
من ذلك ثمّ ينيلونهم الأحساء والأشربة وليس يريد بقراط بهذا القول أنّه ينبغى ٨
أن يغذى جميع المرضى منذ أوّل يوم من المرض لكنّه إنّما يريد أنّه لا ينبغى
أن يغيّر تدبير المريض من المنع من الغذاء إلى التغذّى قبل وقت منتهى المرض
لكن ينبغى أن يحذر فى جميع الأوقات كلّ غذاء خلا كشك الشعير كما قال أوّلا
ويحذر أيضا كشك الشعير فى وقت منتهى المرض وممّا يدلّك على ذلك أنّه بعد هذا ٩
الكلام الذى تقدّم ذكره ذكر أشياء كثيرة من أمر كلّ تغيّر يكون بغتة فى التدبير ثمّ
أتبع ذلك بأن قال هذا القول فى جميع هذه الأشياء التى وصفت أعظم الدلائل على
أنّ تدبير هؤلاء الأطبّاء للمرضى ليس بصواب لكنّهم يستعملون خلاء العروق فى
أمراض لا ينبغى استعماله فيها وهم سيغذون أصحابها بعد بالأحساء ويغيّرون

4 منه] امر B 7 ذلك^I om. B 8 كانت^I] كان B أو] و B 9 إن om. B 10 ante اليوم add. اول B 11 فى^II om. B 12 الحادة om. B 15 يوم من om. B 16 من المنع . . . منتهى المرض om. B 18 يدل B 19 تقدم ذكره] قال B 20 على om. B

be restricted throughout the whole length of their illness to taking
drink, without their being given any food at all, and I myself could
collect enough of his remarks on that point to produce a complete
book. However, I know that if I did, it would bore you and so I will
return to my intended plan and try to carry it out by endeavouring
to produce a reasonably short summary of the whole of Hippocrates' treatment of acute diseases.

I say, then, that in Hippocrates' opinion the doctors who commit 6
the greatest fault are those who make their patients fast for three or
four days at the beginning of their illness and then afterwards proceed
to feed them when the climax is near. For they should either not keep
the patient from food, if his strength is not equal to combatting the
disease, or, if it is, he should be made to fast in accordance with the
regimen imposed on him from the start of his illness until this matures,
if it does so on the fifth, sixth or seventh day. This is Hippocrates'
opinion. As for the theories of other doctors, these can be learnt from 7
his account. He writes in his "On Regimen in Acute Diseases" as
follows: "I know that many doctors do precisely the opposite of what
they should. For they all desiccate the bodies of their patients for two,
three or more days from the start of their illness and then give them
broth and something to drink."[1] Hippocrates does not mean here 8
that all patients should be fed from the first day of their illness, but
only that their treatment should not be changed from fasting to
feeding before the climax. However, one should always be careful of
all kinds of food except barley gruel, as he said at the start, and even
this should be used cautiously at the climax of an illness. Amongst the 9
things which indicate this is the fact that, after the sentence which
I have quoted, Hippocrates goes on to make a number of points
dealing with every sudden change of diet. He follows that by writing:
"In all these details that have been mentioned is the most substantial
evidence that the treatment prescribed by these doctors for their
patients is not correct. Rather, they employ the emptying of the veins
in diseases where it should not be used, when they are about to feed
their patients afterwards on broth, changing the diet and turning

---

[1] *οἶδα δὲ τοὺς ἰητροὺς τὰ ἐναντιώτατα ἢ ὡς δεῖ ποιέοντας· βούλονται γὰρ πάντες ὑπὸ τὰς ἀρχὰς τῶν νούσων προταριχεύσαντες τοὺς ἀνθρώπους ἢ δύο ἢ τρεῖς ἢ καὶ πλείους ἡμέρας οὕτω προσφέρειν τὰ ῥυφήματα καὶ τὰ πόματα.* De diaet. in morb. acut., I 122, 2–6 Kw.

التدبير فينقلونه من خلاء العروق إلى استعمال الأحساء فى أمراض لا ينبغى أن يغيّر
١٠ فيها فدلّ دلالة بيّنة فى هذا القول أنّه قد يكون من الأمراض ما لا ينبغى أن
ينقل تدبير أصحابها من خلاء العروق يعنى من الحمية والمنع من الغذاء إلى
١١ استعمال الأحساء وينبغى أن ننظر ما معنى قوله أن لا ينقل من المنع من الغذاء أمّا أنا
فأرى أنّ ذلك ليس هو شىء غير أن يمنع المريض من الغذاء فى مدّة مرضه كلّها
وذلك أنّه إن كان يذمّ الأطبّاء وينسبهم إلى تعدّى الصواب فى نقلهم تدبير
المريض من المنع من الغذاء إلى التغذية فى بعض الأمراض فهو لا محالة يحمد من
يمنع أصحاب تلك الأمراض من الغذاء إلى أن يأتى البحران وقد صرّح بقراط
بذلك فيما بعد فى هذا القول ثمّ من بعد فلا ينبغى أن تستعمل الأحساء دون أن ينضج
١٢ المرض ما أعجب الرجل الذى هذى فألقى إليك ما ألقى من غير أن يكون عنده
منه علم من الخفّة وضعف الرأى فإنّه لو كان معه شىء من الحزم لقد كان لو لم
يقف على شىء ممّا قرأه فى ذلك الكتاب أعنى كتاب تدبير الأمراض الحادّة
فلا أقلّ من أن كان يقف منه على هذا القول أنّه لا ينبغى أن تستعمل الأحساء دون
أن ينضج المرض يعنى أنّك إذا قدرت فى المريض منذ أوّل مرضه أن تمنعه من
الغذاء ثلاثة أيّام متوالية أو أربعة فلا ينبغى لك أن تنيله شيئا من الأحساء دون أن
١٣ ينضج مرضه إلاّ أن يعرض عارض يضطرّك إلى أن تفعل ذلك فقد أتبع بقراط هذا
القول بأن قال أو تظهر علامة أخرى فى الأمعاء تدلّ على خلاء العروق أو على
١٤ شىء مهيّج وقد دلّ بقراط على رأيه فى تدبير الأمراض الحادّة لا مرّة ولا مرّتين
لكن مرارا كثيرة فى هذا الكتاب الواحد الذى قد يجعل بعضهم رسمه على غير

1 فينقولونه B 2 فدلّ] قبل B 3 يعنى] وتغير B 5 أنّ om. B
شىء sic 7 فهو لا] فهولاء B 8 post يمنع add. من A 10 بالرجل B
هذى فألقى] لغى ما هذا A : تعدا فالقى B : emend. Strohmaier 14 إذا] ان B
18 على om. A 19 بعض B

from emptying the veins to the use of broth in cases where no change should be made."[1]

In this statement Hippocrates shows quite clearly that there are 10
some diseases where one should not change the treatment of the patient from emptying the veins, by which is meant a restrictive diet and prohibition from food, to the use of broth. We must consider, then, what he means when he says that we should not change from a prohibitive diet. In my opinion this can only imply that the patient should 11
be denied food for the whole period of his illness. For if he used to blame doctors and accuse them of overstepping the right course when they switched the treatment of their patients in certain illnesses from a prohibitive diet to the taking of food, he must undoubtedly approve of those who deny them food until the crisis comes. Subsequently he makes this clear enough in the following sentence: "Then broth should not be used unless the disease has matured."[2]

I wonder at the inanity and feeble-mindedness of the man who 12
babbled to you about this without knowing anything about it. For had he any strength of judgement, even if he could understand nothing else of what he read in that book, I mean "On Regimen in Acute Diseases", he should at least have understood this remark in it, that broth should not be used unless the disease has matured. For this means that, when you can keep a patient from food for three or four successive days after the start of his illness, you should not give him any broth until this illness matures, unless some accidental complication ensues which forces you to do that. Hippocrates follows this by 13
saying: "or unless another symptom appears in the intestines which shows clearly that the veins are empty or that there is some irritant."[3]
He has, then, clearly demonstrated his theory about the treatment 14
of acute diseases not once or twice but many times in this one book, which some people have wrongly entitled "Against the Theories of

---

[1] *πάντα οὖν ταῦτα μεγάλα μαρτύρια, ὅτι οὐκ ὀρθῶς ἄγουσιν ἐς τὰ διαιτήματα οἱ ἰητροὶ τοὺς κάμνοντας· ἀλλ' ἐν ᾗσί τε νούσοισιν οὐ χρὴ κενεαγγεῖν τοὺς μέλλοντας ῥυφήμασι διαιτᾶσθαι, κενεαγγέουσιν, ἐν ᾗσί τε οὐ χρὴ μεταβάλλειν ἐκ κενεαγγίης ἐς ῥυφήματα, ἐν ταύτῃσι μεταβάλλουσι.* De diaet. in morb. acut., I 129, 13–18 Kw.

[2] *ἔπειτα οὐ χρηστέον ῥυφήμασιν, πρὶν ἡ νοῦσος πεπανθῇ* De diaet. in morb. acut., I 133, 21 sq. Kw.

[3] *ἢ ἄλλο τι σημεῖον φανῇ ἢ κατὰ ἔντερον, κενεαγγικὸν ἢ ἐρεθιστικόν* De diaet. in morb. acut., I 134, 1 sq. Kw.

الصواب فى المناقضة لآراء أهل قنيدس وبعضهم يجعل رسمه فى كشك الشعير
وذلك أنّه يأمر إمّا بأن لا يغذى المريض بتّة إلى أن ينضج مرضه وإمّا بأن يغذى
منذ أوّل مرضه

٧ وقد قال بقراط فى هذا الكتاب قولا آخر لا أحسب الرجل الذى يكذب
عندك بما يكذب وهذى فهمه عن آخره وهو هذا القول وقد ينبغى فى مواضع كثيرة
أن يدفع الغذاء بتّة وذلك متى كان المريض يحتمل أن يبقى إلى أن يبلغ مرضه منتهاه
وينضج وليس ينبغى أن يتلقّى قول بقراط بمثل فهم ذلك الرجل لكنّه إنّما ينبغى ٢
أن يتلقّى بفهم من قد تعوّد أن يفهم المعانى على حقائقها وقد وصف بقراط هذا
المعنى بلفظ آخر فقال انّه ينبغى أن يتجنّب الغذاء كلّه إلى أن يأتى منتهى المرض
وينضج ووصف هذا المعنى بعينه فى الكلام الذى ذكرته قبيل فقال ثمّ من بعد
فلا ينبغى أن تستعمل الأحساء دون أن ينضج المرض وجملة قول بقراط فى ذلك ٣
أنّه متى كانت حال المريض فى مرضه الحال التى يأتيه معها البحران نحو اليوم
الخامس ثمّ امتنع من الغذاء فى الأيّام الثلاثة الأول من مرضه واغتذى فى اليوم
الرابع ناله من ذلك ضرر عظيم جدّا والذى يراه بقراط ضدّ هذا أعنى أنّه إن كان
المريض قويّا فلا ينبغى أن يغذى بتّة قبل اليوم الخامس وإن كان ضعيفا
فينبغى أن يغذى فى الأوّل إلى الرابع بماء الشعير ثمّ يكون ما يغتذى به منه فى
اليوم الرابع أقلّ ممّا كان يغتذى به منه فى الأيّام التى قبله ثمّ يمسك عن الغذاء فى
اليوم الخامس وذلك أيضا يضح لك ويتبيّن إن أنت قرأت الكلام الذى وضعت منه ٤
قبيل حرفا عن آخره وهو هذا فى جميع هذه الأشياء التى وصفت أعظم الدلائل على
أنّ تدبير هؤلاء الأطبّاء للمرضى ليس بصواب لكنّهم يستعملون خلاء العروق
فى أمراض لا ينبغى استعماله فيها وهم سيغذون أصحابها بعد بالأحساء ويغيّرون
التدبير وينقلونه من خلاء العروق إلى استعمال الأحساء فى أمراض لا ينبغى أن يغيّر

1 لآراء] لان B   2 إلى أن ينضج مرضه *om.* B   3 منذ] من B   7 و^II *om.* B
ذلك *om.* B   8 قد^I *om.* B   10 ذكرته] وصفته B   13 اليوم *om.* B
14 يراه] يريد B   15 يغتذى B   16 يغذى] يغتذى B   *post* فى^I *add.* الايام B
18 ايضا يضح] انما يصح B   17 يمسك] يسد B   ثمّ يكون ما] ويكون B
20 الاطبّاء للمرضى] المرضى B   19 وفى B   منه *om.* B   وضعت] وصفت B

the School of Cnidus", and others "On Barley Gruel."[1] For he recommends that the patient should either not be fed at all until his disease matures, or else that he should be fed from the start of it.

7. In this book Hippocrates makes another remark which I do not think was fully grasped by the man who told you those senseless lies. It runs as follows: "In many cases food should not be given at all, that is, where the patient is able to endure until his disease reaches its climax and matures."[2] One should not apply to these remarks your 2
informant's type of understanding but rather that of a man who is accustomed to grasping the real significance of ideas. It is the same notion that has been expressed by Hippocrates in other words where he says that all food should be avoided until the disease reaches its climax and matures. The passage which I quoted shortly before this contains the same idea. It ran: "Then broth should not be used unless the disease has matured."[3]

Hippocrates' point may be summarised as follows. When the 3
patient's condition is such that his crisis will arrive towards the fifth day and he is then denied food for the first three days and fed on the fourth day, he will suffer very great harm through this treatment. What Hippocrates thought should be done is the opposite of this – I mean that, if the patient is strong, he should not be fed at all before the fifth day. If he is weak, from the first to the fourth day he should be fed on barley water and the quantity of this given him on the fourth day should be less than that given on the previous days. Afterwards, on the fifth day he should be kept from food. You can see this 4
clearly enough if you read in full the passage from which I quoted a section shortly before this. It runs as follows: "In all these details that have been mentioned is the most substantial evidence that the treatment prescribed by these doctors for their patients is not correct. Rather, they employ the emptying of the veins in diseases where this should not be used, when they are about to feed their patients afterwards on broth, changing the diet and turning from the emptying of the veins to the use of broth in cases where no change should be made.

---

[1] *τοῦτον τὸν λόγον ἀναγνῶναί μοι δοκοῦσι μόνον οἱ Περὶ πτισάνης ἐπιγράψαντες τὸ βιβλίον, ὥσπερ αὖ πάλιν οἱ Πρὸς τὰς Κνιδίας γνώμας τὸ πρῶτον προοίμιον·* CMG V 9, 1 p. 133, 23–25.

[2] *τὴν ἀφαίρεσιν ὅλως ἀφελεῖν πολλαχοῦ λυσιτελεῖ, ὅπου διαρκεῖν μέλλει ὁ κάμνων, μέχρι ἂν τῆς νούσου ἡ ἀκμὴ πεπανθῇ.* De diaet. in morb. acut., I 127, 19–21 Kw.

[3] De diaet. in morb. acut., I 133, 21 sq. Kw. loc. cit.

فيها وهم فى أكثر الأمر من ذلك على خطاء وذلك أنّهم كانوا كثيرا ما ينقلون
المريض من خلاء العروق إلى استعمال الأحساء فى الأوقات التى ينتفع فيها كثيرا
بالنقلة من الأحساء إلى المشارفة لخلاء العروق إن اتّفق أن يكون استصعاب
المرض فى ذلك الوقت أفلا ترى أنّ بقراط يأمر أن يستعمل فى منتهى المرض خلاء ٥
العروق ويعنى به الامتناع من الغذاء فالرجل إذًا الذى ظنّ بابقراط أنّه يأمر بأن
يغذى المريض فى كلّ يوم مستحقّ للذمّ وذلك أنّه معما أخطأ فيه من جميع
ما ادّعاه على بقراط قد أخطأ أيضا فى هذا المعنى الذى وصفته الآن وذلك أنّ بقراط
وإن غذا المريض فى سائر الأيّام المتقدّمة بالحذر منه أن تسقط قوّته فإنّه عند
منتهى مرضه يمنعه من الغذاء فيجب من هذا ألّا يوجد مرض من الأمراض يغذو
فيه بقراط صاحبه فى جميع الأيّام إلّا أن يكون صاحب المرض فى غاية الضعف
وإذا كان ذلك كذلك فليس يمكن أن يحتمل المرض الحادّ أصلا

٨ وهذه الشهادة كلّها إنّما أتيتك بها منّ كتاب بقراط فى تدبير الأمراض الحادّة
وليس من كلّ ذلك الكتاب لكن من النصف منه لأنّ النصف الآخر الباقى قد يقال
إنّه ليس هو لابقراط فإن نظرت فيما ذكره فى كتاب الفصول فى هذا الباب وجدت ٢
معناه فيه ومعناه فى كتاب تدبير الأمراض الحادّة معنى واحدا وبعض قوله فى هذا
الباب فى كتاب الفصول هو هذا وإذا كان المرض حادّا جدّا فإنّ الأوجاع
التى فى الغاية القصوى تأتى فيه بدءا ويجب ضرورة أن تستعمل فيه ألطف التدبير
الذى هو فى الغاية القصوى من اللطافة فأىّ التدبير عندك هو ألطف التدبير الذى ٣
هو فى الغاية القصوى التدبير الذى يغذى فيه المريض فى كلّ يوم أو التدبير الذى هو

1 كانوا om. B 2 من] فى B 5 و om. B 6 للذمّ] لان يذم B
معما] ما B 7 المعنى] الكلام B 8 فى] من B 11 ذلك om. B
أصلا om. B 12 و om. B 13 منه om. B الآخر om. B 16 وهو B
17 ألطف om. A 18 sq. ألطف . . . هو] الاولى والاشبه بالتدبير الذى B

Here, for the most part, they are at fault in that they often alter their patient's treatment from the emptying of the veins to the use of broth at times when there would be considerable benefit in making the opposite change to something approximating the emptying of the veins, should the disease then have become aggravated."[1]

Hippocrates, you see, recommends emptying the veins, by which 5
he means abstention from food, at the climax of the disease. As this is so, the man who thought that he was recommending us to feed the patient daily deserves to be censured. For here too, on the point that I have just described, he has added a further mistake to the others that he has made in his Hippocratic claims. For even if Hippocrates feeds a patient through all the rest of the initial period of his illness to guard against a failure of his strength, at the climax he keeps him from food. It must follow, then, that there is no single disease where he feeds his patient every day, except in cases of extreme weakness, and there the patient will not be able to support an acute disease at all.

8. All this evidence I am producing for you only from Hippocrates' "On Regimen in Acute Diseases". Nor is it taken from the whole of this work, but only from half of it, as the other, the remaining, half is said not to have been written by Hippocrates[2]. If you look 2
at his remarks on this point in the "Aphorisms" you will find that they coincide precisely with his theories in the "Regimen in Acute Diseases". For amongst his statements on this in the "Aphorisms" is the following: "When the disease is very acute, it is immediately attended by extremely violent pains and one must employ in its treatment a regimen that reaches the extreme of lightness."[3] Which regimen, then, do you 3
think is the one which reaches the extreme of lightness – the one where the patient is fed every day or its opposite, I mean the one

---

[1] *πάντα οὖν ταῦτα μεγάλα μαρτύρια, ὅτι οὐκ ὀρθῶς ἄγουσιν ἐς τὰ διαιτήματα οἱ ἰητροὶ τοὺς κάμνοντας· ἀλλ' ἐν ᾗσί τε νούσοισιν οὐ χρὴ κενεαγγεῖν τοὺς μέλλοντας ῥυφήμασι διαιτᾶσθαι, κενεαγγέουσιν, ἐν ᾗσί τε οὐ χρὴ μεταβάλλειν ἐκ κενεαγγίης ἐς ῥυφήματα, ἐν ταύτῃσι μεταβάλλουσι. καὶ ὡς ἐπὶ τὸ πολὺ ἀπαρτὶ ἐν τούτοισι τοῖσι καιροῖσι μεταβάλλουσιν ἐς τὰ ῥυφήματα ἐκ τῆς κενεαγγίης, ἐν οἷσι πολλάκις ἀρήγει ἐκ τῶν ῥυφημάτων πλησιάζειν τῇ κενεαγγίῃ, ἢν οὕτω τύχῃ παροξυνομένη ἡ νοῦσος.* De diaet. in morb. acut., I 129, 13–22 Kw.

[2] *ἐν τῷ Περὶ διαίτης τὰ μετὰ τὸν περὶ τοῦ λουτροῦ λόγον εἰρημένα προσηκόντως ὑπώπτευσαν οὐκ ὀλίγοι τῶν ἰατρῶν ὡς οὐχ Ἱπποκράτους ὄντα·* CMG V 9, 1 p. 271, 3–5.

[3] Aphor. I 7 *ὅκου μὲν κάτοξυ τὸ νούσημα, αὐτίκα καὶ τοὺς ἐσχάτους πόνους ἔχει, καὶ τῇ ἐσχάτως λεπτοτάτῃ διαίτῃ ἀναγκαῖον χρέεσθαι·* (IV 462, 12sq. L.).

على ضدّ ذلك أعنى الذى لا يغذى فيه المريض بتّة فإنّ هذه اللفظة أعنى قوله
ألطف التدبير هى من الألفاظ التى يسمّيها أصحاب النحو من اليونانيّين ألفاظ
الإغراق وهى أن تضع الشىء فى غاية ما يمكن أن يبلغه حتّى لا يوجد فى جنسه
شىء يفوقه فإن أنت وضعت أنّ مريضا مرض سبعة أيّام وكان فى كلّ ٤
يوم من تلك الأيّام يغتذى بغذاء لم يجز لأحد أن يقول فيه انّه مدبّر بألطف
التدبير لأنّ الذى ترك الغذاء يوما واحداً من تلك الأيّام السبعة ألطف تدبيرا
منه والذى امتنع من الغذاء أيضا يومين ألطف تدبيرا من تدبير الثانى والذى ترك
الغذاء ثلاثة أيّام ألطف تدبيرا من الثالث والذى تركه أربعة أيّام ألطف تدبيرا من
الرابع والذى تركه خمسة أيّام ألطف تدبيرا من الخامس والذى تركه ستّة
أيّام ألطف تدبيرا من السادس والذى امتنع من الغذاء سبعة أيّام فهو ألطف
تدبيرا من السابع وليس يمكن أن يكون أحد ألطف تدبيرا من هذا فالذى مدبّر ٥
إذاً بألطف التدبير إنّما هو هذا الذى امتنع من الغذاء أيّام مرضه كلّها إلى أن
جاز منتهى المرض ويدلّك على أنّ هذا المعنى هو معنى بقراط الزيادة التى
زادها فقال الذى فى الغاية القصوى من اللطافة وذلك أنّه لم يكتف بأن يقول انّه ٦
يجب أن يستعمل ألطف التدبير فى صاحب المرض الذى فى غاية الحدّة على
أنّه ليس بعد ألطف التدبير غاية أخرى من اللطافة لكنّه زاد فى قوله الذى
فى الغاية القصوى من اللطافة واحتمل أن يكون معنى واحد مرّتين كيما يبيّن معناه
ويشرحه فإنّ البلوغ إلى الغاية قد يدلّ عليه قوله ألطف التدبير ويدلّ عليه أيضا
قوله الذى فى الغاية القصوى من اللطافة وعلى هذا القياس فقد كان يكتفى بإحدى ٧
اللفظتين لكنّه إنّما استعملهما جميعا وهو يريد أن يدلّ أنّه ليس من ماء
الشعير فقط يمنع من كان مرضه بتلك الحال لكن قد يمنعه أيضا من ماء العسل فإنّ
الاقتصار بالمريض على ماء العسل من ألطف التدبير إلّا أنّه وإن كان كذلك
فليس هو من ألطف التدبير الذى فى الغاية القصوى فلمّا زاد فى قوله الذى فى ٨
الغاية القصوى كان المعنى الّذى يشير إليه فيه هو المعنى الذى يثلب به ارسسطراطس

1 البتة B 2 التى . . . الفاظ *om.* B 4 وان B 5 بغذاء *om.* B يدبر B 6 الذى] اخر B 8 تدبيرا . . . من الثالث *om.* B 9 sq. من . . . الخامس *om.* B 11 أحد] اجزا B يدبر B 13 المرض] مرضه B المعنى *om.* B 17 يكون] *fort.* يكرّر *scribendum est* 19 فقد *om.* B 21 تلك B 24 غاية B فيه] بقراط B يثلب] يثبت B

where he is not fed at all? For this expression, I mean the phrase,
"the lightest of regimens", is what is known to Greek grammarians as
a term of hyperbole, the implication being that something has reached
its furthest possible point and that there is nothing in its class which
surpasses it. Think, then, of a sick man whose disease lasts seven days. 4
If he is fed on each of these days, no one can say that he is being
treated with the lightest possible regimen, since whoever abstained
from food on one of the seven would have a lighter regimen. If an-
other man abstained from food for two days, his regimen would be
lighter than the second; if another abstained for three days, this would
be lighter than the third; if another abstained for four days, it would
be lighter than the fourth; if another abstained for five days, it would
be lighter than the fifth; if another abstained for six days, it would be
lighter than the sixth and if another abstained from food for seven
days, then this regimen would be lighter than the seventh and nobody
could be treated with one lighter than it.

Consequently, the patient whose treatment is the lightest of all is 5
the one who is kept from food throughout the whole period of his
illness until the climax has past. That this is what Hippocrates meant
is shown you by what he added to his phrase when he wrote, "that
reaches the extreme of lightness". For he did not confine himself to 6
saying that we should use the lightest regimen for those who suffer
from the most acute diseases, although nothing can be lighter than the
lightest. Rather, he added, "that reaches the extreme of lightness",
and he took it upon himself to repeat the same thing twice in order to
clarify and explain his meaning. For the superlative sense is shown
by the words, "the lightest of diets", and also by the phrase, "that has
reached the extreme of lightness". He could thus have contented him- 7
self by using only one of these two modes of expression. But, in fact,
he used them both since his intention was to show that those who
suffer from illnesses of this kind should be denied not only barley
water but honey water as well. Admittedly, to confine a patient to
honey water is to treat him with a very light regimen, but even at
that it does not represent the lightest regimen which has reached the 8
extreme of lightness. When he adds, "the extreme of lightness", the
point that he is indicating is the one on which Erasistratus blamed

دكسبس وابلونيس تلميذى بقراط أنّهما لم يكونا يقتصران على أن يمنعا المرضى
من جميع الأشياء حتّى كانا يمنعان مع ذلك من الماء والأجود فيما أحسب أن ٩
أضع كلام ارسسطراطس فى ذلك بلفظه وهو هذا فقد يذكرون أنّ ابلونيس
ودكسبس تلميذا بقراط اللذان أخذا عنه كانا يهيّئان مكاييل من شمع يكون اثنا
عشر منها سدس رطل ويكيلون للمريض بتلك المكاييل من الماء فى اليوم ثلاثة
وكانا فى سائر تدبيرهم للمرضى يحصرانهم الحصر الشديد ويضيّقان عليهم
ولا يدعانهم يرزؤون شيئا بتّة لأنّهما كانا يريان أنّ كلّ رطوبة ينالها المريض
إنّما تصير مادّة لحمّاه بمنزلة الوقود لها فهذا قول ارسسطراطس فى أنّ تلميذى ١٠
بقراط كانا يدبّران المرضى بغاية التدبير اللطيف حتّى أنّهما لم يكونا ينيلانهم من
الماء مقدار الكفاية فضلا عن كلّ شىء وصاحبك هذا يتضمّن من الخبر برأى بقراط ما
يفوق فيه ارسسطراطس وتلميذى بقراط ثمّ عمد إلى كلام من كلام بقراط أخرجه ١١
لك يستشهد به على صحّة ما ذكر فقطع بعضه عن كلام يتّصل به فيه تمام معناه
وأسقط من بعضه ما لا يتمّ المعنى إلّا به وغيّر بعضه وقطع أوائل بعضه ثمّ ذمّ
أهل هذا الدهر من الأطبّاء ونسبهم إلى أنّهم يقتلون الناس من الجوع وحمد بقراط
على أنّه كان يشبع المريض كلّ يوم بزعمه وبقراط يبلغ من تدقيقه لتدبير المرضى ١٢
أن لم يعط أحدا منهم الحسو المتّخذ من الحنطة التى يقال لها خندروس فضلا عن
سائر الأطعمة التى يعطيها جميع المرضى † إلّا الخطاء † فى دهرنا هذا

1 دكسبس] لاوركسيس B 3 بلفظه *om.* B 4 تلميذى B اللذين B
6 عليهم *om.* B 10 مقدار الكفاية *post* كل شىء *trsp.* B 11 يفوق فيه] هو فيه فوق B ثم عمد إلى كلام] ويحكى لك كلاما B 16 انه B الخندرس B
17 إلّا الخطاء] *fort.* الأطبّاء *scribendum est*

his pupils, Dexippus and Apollonius, in that they did not confine themselves to denying their patients everything else, but they even prevented them from drinking water.

My best course, I think, is to quote word for word what Erasistra- 9
tus said on that point. For he wrote: "They say that Apollonius and Dexippus, pupils of Hippocrates, who studied under him, used to prepare wax measures, twelve of which held one sixth of a *raṭl* and they would daily ladle out three of these measures full of water to their patients. For the rest, in their regimen they employed very severe restrictions and did not allow their patients to get anything to eat at all. For they thought that whatever moisture the patient received served like fuel as material for his fever."[1]

This, then, is what Erasistratus said, to the effect that the two 10
pupils of Hippocrates used to treat their patients with the lightest of regimens, to such an extent that they did not allow them a sufficiency of water, let alone anything else. But this friend of yours has more information about Hippocrates' theories than had Erasistratus and Hippocrates' pupils. He then betakes himself to words 11
of Hippocrates which he produces for you in order to prove the truth of what he has to say. He divorces some of them from the context which gives them their full meaning; from some he leaves out what is necessary to complete the sense; another phrase he alters and he cuts the beginning from another[2]. Then he criticises our contemporary doctors and accuses them of killing their patients by hunger and he praises Hippocrates on the ground that he used to give his their fill to eat each day – as he thinks. Yet Hippocrates takes the refine- 12
ment of his patients' regimen so far that he gives none of them broth made from the so-called *χόνδρος* wheat, let alone any of the other dishes which all the sick ... are given in this age of ours.

---

[1] *τοὺς μαθητὰς αὐτοῦ* (sc. *Ἱπποκράτους*) *δῆθεν μεμφόμενος Ἀπολλώνιόν τε καὶ Δέξιππον, οὕς φησι, κηρίνους κυάθους δώδεκα ποιήσαντας εἰς τὸν ἑκτημορίτην τῆς κοτύλης κύαθον, ἕνα τούτων ἢ δύο ἀπομετρεῖν τοῖς πυρέττουσιν·* CMG V 9, 1 p. 256, 2–5; cf. 277, 3 sqq.

[2] Cf.: *καὶ ταύτην τὴν ῥῆσιν ὁ δοὺς ἰατρὸς Βίκτωρι τῷ Ῥώμης ἐπάρχῳ τὸ Περὶ τῆς καθ' Ἱπποκράτην διαίτης καὶ ἄλλας τινὰς ἐξ ἡμισείας ἐνέγραψε τῷ βιβλίῳ, καθάπερ κἀκείνην ἐν ᾗ φησιν "ὅτι οὐ στερητέαι αἱ πρῶται ἡμέραι τοῦ ῥοφήματος", ἔτι δὲ πρὸς αὐτῇ "καὶ τοῖσι μέν γε εἰθισμένοισι δὶς σιτεῖσθαι τῆς ἡμέρης δὶς δοτέον". ἀλλὰ τούτων μὲν τῶν δύο ῥήσεων ἑκατέρας ἀφεῖλε τὸ ἥμισυ μέρος, τῆς δὲ νῦν προκειμένης ἀφεῖλε μὲν οὐδέν, οὐ προσέθηκε δὲ τὸν καιρόν,* CMG V 9, 1 p. 265, 22–266, 1.

٩ ولكنّه يحتجّ فيقول انّ تلك الحنطة لم تكن عرفت بعد فى ذلك الدهر ولو
كانت عرفت لقد كان بقراط لا محالة يستعملها ويشبه هؤلاء الأطبّاء أن يقولوا
مثل هذا القول انّ القدماء من شعراء اليونانيّين لم يذكروا هذه الحنطة ولا ذكرها بقراط
فى شىء من المقالات الثلاثة التى له فى التدبير إلّا أنّ صاحبك يقول انّ ذلك
الكتاب ليس هو لبقراط فإن شئت فاجعل ذلك الكتاب لفيلسطيون وإن شئت
فاجعله لارسطن وإن شئت فاجعله لفانطس فما من هؤلاء أحد إلّا قديم ولم يكن بحثنا ٢
هل ذلك الكتاب لابقراط بالحقيقة أم لا وإنّما كان البحث هل كانت تلك
الحنطة التى ذكرنا فى ذلك الدهر أم لا وإنّما حملت إلينا الآن قريبا من بلاد
الهند أو من بلاد الأتراك الذين فى أقصى الشمال فكان ذلك الكتاب لابقراط أو
كان لفيليسطيون أوكان لأرسطون أوكان لفانطس فقد بان ووضح ما قصدنا
إليه وتبيّن أيضا من أنّ القدماء من شعراء اليونانيّين يذكرون تلك الحنطة وقد ذكرها ٣
أيضا الرجل الذى كتب المقالة الصغرى من المقالتين اللتين فى العلل المنسوبتين إلى
ابقراط كان ذلك الرجل فولوبس وهو أشهر تلامذة ابقراط أوكان اعروفن وهو أيضا
رجل نبيه كان على عهد ابقراط ولست أضايق فى هذا لكنّى أسلّم أنّ ابقراط لم ٤
يعرف تلك الحنطة إلّا أنّى أقول إنّه لا بدّ من أن يكون الخبز قد كان عرف فى ذلك
الوقت فما بال ابقراط لا يستعمل الخبز فى الكتاب الذى وصف فيه تدبير أصحاب
الأمراض الحادّة أمّا أنا فالجواب عندى فى هذا أسهل وأنتزعه من نصّ كلام ٥
بقراط حين قال إنّ كشك الشعير عندى بالصواب اختير على سائر الأغذية التى

6 فاجعله . . . لارسطن *om.* B   أحد] أيضا B   ولم يكن] فيكون B
8 بلاد *om.* B   10 كان^I] شئت B   11 أنّ *om.* B   13 أو] و B
13 اعروفن] اوروفن B   و^II *om.* B   14 على *om.* B   17 نصّ] فص B

9. However, your friend argues that this type of wheat was not yet
known in Hippocrates' time and, if it had been, he would undoubt-
edly have used it. It seems that the same point is made by these doc-
tors who claim that this wheat is not mentioned by the old Greek
poets or by Hippocrates in any of the three tracts that he wrote on
regimen. Your friend of course, claims that that work is not by Hippo-
crates and, if you like, you can take its author as Philistion or
Ariston or Phaon. All of them, without exception, are ancient[1].
Here, however, we are not concerned to enquire whether, in fact, it 2
was written by Hippocrates or not. We are dealing only with the
question whether the grain mentioned was known then or not, or
whether it has only quite recently been imported to us from India or
from the land of the Turks in the far north[2]. So whether that book
is by Hippocrates, Philistion, Ariston or Phaon, the point
which we wish to make is, nevertheless, plain and obvious. Actually, 3
it is also made clear enough by the fact that the old Greek poets[3]
do mention that grain and it is noted as well by the writer of the shorter
of the two tracts on illnesses, both of which are attributed to Hippo-
crates. The author is either Polybus, the most famous of Hippo-
crates' pupils, or Euryphon, who was also a famous man and a
contemporary of Hippocrates. However, I do not press this point 4
and I will concede that Hippocrates did not know of that grain.
I would point out, however, that bread must have been known in his
time. Why, then, does he make no use of it in the book where he
describes regimen in acute diseases? I have an easy answer to this, 5
which I take from the actual text of Hippocrates' remarks. He
writes: "In these diseases barley gruel is in my opinion rightly pre-
ferred to anything else that is made of grain. I commend those who do

---

[1] Cf.: *τοὺς γὰρ οἰομένους μηδέπω χόνδρον εἶναι κατὰ τοὺς Ἱπποκράτους χρόνους ἀγνοοῦντας ἐλέγξεις ἐκ τοῦ τῶν παλαιῶν κωμικῶν ἐνίους ἐμνημονευκέναι χόνδρου, καὶ αὐτὸν δὲ τὸν Ἱπποκράτην ἐν τῷ Περὶ διαίτης ὑγιεινῷ. εἰ γὰρ καὶ μὴ Ἱπποκράτους ἐστὶν ἐκεῖνο τὸ βιβλίον, ἀλλ' Εὐρυφῶντος ἢ Φαῶντος ἢ Φιλιστίωνος ἢ Ἀρίστωνος ἢ τινος ἄλλου τῶν παλαιῶν (εἰς πολλοὺς γὰρ ἀναφέρουσιν αὐτό), πάντες ἐκεῖνοι τῶν παλαιῶν ἀνδρῶν εἰσιν* CMG V 9, 1 p. 134, 33–135, 5.

[2] Strohmaier identifies this with Scythia, v. Hippocrates, De aere, aquis et locis (CMG I 1 p. 71, 12sqq.) and the Arabic translation in Aya Sofya 3632 (fol. 54^v 18sqq.).

[3] Cf. J. M. Edmonds, The Fragments of the Attic Comedy, vol. 1, Leiden 1957, p. 246 (fragm. 108, l. 18 Pherecrates), p. 632, 690 (fragm. 203, 412 Aristophanes).

تتّخذ من الحبوب فى هذه الأمراض وأحمد من لا يذمّه واختاره على غيره وذلك لأنّ فيه لزوجة معها ملاسة واتّصال ولين وزلق ورطوبة معتدلة وتسكين للعطش وسرعة انغسال إن احتيج إلى ذلك أيضا منه وليس فيه قبض ولا تهيّج ردىء ولا ينتفخ ويربو فى المعدة لأنّه قد انتفخ وربا فى الطبخ غاية ما كان يمكن فيه أن ينتفخ ويربو فى هذه الوجوه وفى وجوه أخر شبيهة بها يحمد ابقراط فيها كشك الشعير ٦ وليس يوجد فى غيره من سائر الأغذية نصف هذه المنافع فضلا عن كلّها ولذلك اقتصر ابقراط على كشك الشعير فى تدبير أصحاب الأمراض الحادّة

1 لا om. B 4 ويربو] ولا يربو A 5 فيها] فيما بعد B 6 هذه] تلك B
7 in fine add. تم كتاب جالينوس فى تدبير الامراض الحادة على راى ابقراط ترجمة حنين بن اسحق المتطبب ولله الحمد كثيرا A: تم الكتاب باسره والحمد لله رب العلمين (sic) B

not find fault with it, using it in preference to other dishes. For its ingredients are viscous, smooth, interconnected, soft and slippery. It contains a moderate amount of moisture and can be used to quench thirst, and it can quickly be purged away, if that too happens to be necessary. It has no astringency or any unpleasant irritant quality, nor does it expand and swell in the stomach, since it has already expanded as much as it can in the process of being cooked."[1]

Hippocrates, then, praises barley gruel on these counts and on 6
others like them, nor is any other foodstuff found to possess the half of these advantages, let alone the whole of them. For that reason Hippocrates confines himself to barley gruel in his treatment of those suffering from acute diseases.

---

[1] *πτισάνη μὲν οὖν δοκεῖ ὀρθῶς προκεκρίσθαι τῶν σιτηρῶν γευμάτων ἐν τούτοισι τοῖσι νοσήμασιν, καὶ ἐπαινέω τοὺς προκρίναντας. τὸ γὰρ γλίσχρασμα αὐτῆς λεῖον καὶ συνεχὲς καὶ προσηνές ἐστι καὶ ὀλισθηρὸν καὶ πλαδαρὸν μετρίως καὶ ἄδιψον καὶ εὐέκκριτον (εὐέκπλυτον* Ḥunain), *εἴ τι καὶ τούτου προσδέοι, καὶ οὔτε στύψιν ἔχον οὔτε ἄραδον κακὸν οὔτε ὀνοιδίσκεται ἐν τῇ κοιλίῃ· ἀνῴδηκε γὰρ ἐν τῇ ἑψήσει, ὅσον πλεῖστον ἐπεφύκει διογκοῦσθαι.* De diaet. in morb. acut., I 113, 19–114, 5 Kw.

THE LATIN VERSIONS OF

DE PARTIBVS ARTIS MEDICATIVAE

AND

DE CAVSIS CONTENTIVIS

PRAEMONITUM

Es mag den einen oder anderen Benutzer befremden, wenn in einem Bande des Supplementum Orientale neben dem arabischen Text auch eine lateinische Edition vorgelegt wird. Doch dürfte dieses Verfahren in dem hier vorliegenden Fall durchaus gerechtfertigt sein.

Von den beiden im griechischen Original verlorengegangenen Galenschriften De partibus artis medicativae und De causis contentivis sind uns lateinische Interlinearübersetzungen überliefert, die von dem bekannten Galenübersetzer Nicolaus von Rhegium (14. Jh.) stammen. Sie wurden von Hermann Schöne (Galenus, De partibus artis medicativae, Greifswald 1911) und Karl Kalbfleisch (Galeni De causis continentibus libellus, Marburg 1904) ediert. Diese beiden Ausgaben sind seit langem vergriffen, und so schien es angezeigt, sie hier erneut zugänglich zu machen, um auf diese Weise dem Benutzer den Vergleich der arabischen und lateinischen Textfassungen zu erleichtern.

Da seit den Editionen von Kalbfleisch und Schöne keine weiteren Handschriften mit dem Text der beiden Schriften bekannt geworden sind, wurde davon abgesehen, eine Neubearbeitung der in ihrem Wert unbestrittenen älteren Ausgaben vorzunehmen. Es wurde lediglich versucht, mit Hilfe der arabischen Überlieferung an einigen Stellen über den bisher vorliegenden Text hinauszukommen oder Konjekturen der Herausgeber zu bestätigen. Ferner wurden die Textvorschläge von Karl Deichgräber (Die griechische Empirikerschule, Berlin 1930, S. 119 bis 121, 140f. u. 154) berücksichtigt. Da die hier vorgelegten Texte, wie dargelegt wurde, die älteren Ausgaben in keiner Weise ersetzen wollen, glaubten wir darauf verzichten zu können, ihre textkritischen Apparate vollständig abzudrucken.

Wir beschränken uns in dem von uns gegebenen kritischen Apparat auf solche Angaben, die entweder zur Erklärung der Zeichen im Text unbedingt erforderlich sind oder sich aus der Einbeziehung der arabischen Übersetzung als Textzeugen ergeben. Um den Apparat weiterhin zu entlasten, werden Textabweichungen, soweit man von ihnen annehmen darf, daß sie auf die Vorlage des arabischen bzw. lateinischen Übersetzers zurückgehen, nicht im Apparat erwähnt, sondern nur in der englischen Übersetzung und in der lateinischen Fassung durch Kursivdruck hervorgehoben. Textausfälle bzw. -zusätze in der arabischen Übersetzung werden ebenfalls durch Kursivdruck in der englischen bzw. lateinischen Übersetzung gekennzeichnet, außerdem jedoch im kritischen Apparat notiert. Von Textergänzungen und der Markierung von Lücken im lateinischen Text wird bis auf wenige Ausnahmen abgesehen, da es in den meisten Fällen nicht definitiv zu entscheiden ist, ob die durch Schreiberversehen entstandenen Textausfälle zu Lasten der lateinischen Überlieferung gehen oder bereits in der griechischen Tradition erfolgten. Gänzlich unberücksichtigt bleiben solche Zusätze im arabischen bzw. lateinischen Text, die sich mit einiger Sicherheit als Interpretament des jeweiligen Übersetzers erkennen lassen.

J. Kollesch, D. Nickel, G. Strohmaier

Berlin, August 1966

GALIENI

DE PARTIBVS ARTIS MEDICATIVAE

CONSPECTVS SIGLORVM

A = Galeni Opera, Venetiis 1490, t. I
B = Galeni Opera, Venetiis 1541

GALIENI

DE PARTIBVS ARTIS MEDICATIVE

1. De partibus medicatiue, Juste dilectissime, conuenienter mihi 7 Schöne
videris dubitare, cum *alii* [et alii] aliter eas distinguant. audire namque 2
est aliquos quidem in *farmaciam* et *cirurgiam* et dietam | totam artem 10
incidentes, deinde rursus unamquamque *predictarum* partium diuiden-
tes, non tamen *simpliciter omnes*. et aliquos in curatiuam et *vocatam*
sanatiuam; alios autem, qui deposcunt et precustoditiuam his adici
mox in prima diuisione, sicut et alii resumptiuam; alii autem utrasque
has et cum istis euecticam. | sunt autem alii, qui et cirocomicam siue 3 15
senum educatiuam sicut propriam quandam partem artis adiciunt
predictis; quidam autem et pedotroficam, id est infantium ⟨educa-
tiuam⟩, sicut et alii decoratiuam et distinguentes eam a commotica.
quidam autem, amplius adhuc diuidentes cum predictis partibus 4
aliam partem paruam mox in | prima connumerant diuisione, vocita- 20
tiuam, alii quidem simpliciter et indeterminate, alii vero cum eo quod
determinant et ostendunt tum quidem eis *qui ad* ⟨. . .⟩ *idoneam*, tum
etiam eis qui secundum naturam se volunt habere, ut sicut [volunt
habere] alios actus, ita habeant et vocem. sed hii quidem nunquam 5
peruenient ut vnicuique eorum, | qui secundum ⟨partes corporis actuum 25
propriam attribuant⟩ partem artis. et siquidem ita fecissent, haberet
aliquam rationem diuisio eorum; sed quia omnes alios relinquunt,
vnius vero solius faciunt memoriam, manifeste redarguunt se ipsos,
quod amethodice et absque ratione faciunt diuisionem. a[u]t neque
⟨qui⟩ per maximas partes pertransierunt, | concordant adinuicem de 30

4 et alii *seclusimus* 12 educatiuam *add.* Schöne 17 *lacunam statuit* Schöne: attempts at voice production may be suitable from the point of view of competition — that is for those who wish to surpass others in this *vers. Arab.* 18 sq. volunt habere *sec. versionem Arabicam seclusimus* 20 sq. partes corporis actuum propriam attribuant *sec. versionem Arabicam addidimus*: naturam actuum propriam attribuant *add.* Schöne

6 harum ipsarum diuisione ad minores partes. alii autem, quedam quidem predictorum ponentes ut partes, non pauca aut⟨em⟩ obmittentes, superaddunt eis alias secundum primam mox diuisionem, sicut qui dixerunt phisiologi⟨c⟩am et passiologicam. alii autem dicunt et materialem simul cum istis, sicut et alii signi|ficatiuam, alii autem causiologicam.

38 2. Emperici autem, fere omnes concordantes adinu⟨i⟩cem in faciendo partium artis duplicem primam et secundum genus diffe|rentiam, alias autem earum finales, alias vero constitutiuas dicentes esse, non concordant adinuicem in harum ipsarum connumeratione. quidam enim eorum finales dixerunt esse signatiuam et curatiuam; alii vero et vocatam sanatiuam, alii autem et decoratiuam, alii autem et voc⟨it⟩atiuam eis ad⟨d⟩iderunt. in constitutiuis vero per | se inspectionem quidem et hystoriam vniuersi, similis vero transitionem non
2 omnes enunciauerunt esse partem artis. at vero neque ⟨in⟩ incidendo singulam predictarum adhuc in minores particulas concordant adinuicem, ut est dicere, emperici et dogmatici; quin etiam, si quidem omnia talia nominauerit aliquis partes medicatiue, qualia | in Roma maxime et ad multa et minora diuidere ea non cessant, dentales quosdam et auriculares et anales medicos nominantes, in aporiam veniet sermo maiorem, quamuis et his occasionem aliquam circa hoc prebuerit nomen optalmicorum, id est oculicorum, non nuper impositum, sed multo iam elapso tempore; si enim oculorum solorum | fuerit aliquis medicus, non irrationabiliter videbitur et dentium aliquis alius esse et alius aurium ⟨et alius⟩ vniuscuiusque corporis partium proprius, ut sint tot medici quot particule, ac etiam apunctores et erniarum incisores alii quidam et lapidum incisores. qui si sic nominentur, plures erunt quam corporis particule medici; secundum | enim
3 vnamquamque passionem erit vnus medicus. et non est mirabile, si in tot multa diuidatur ars maxima existens *et in maxima ciuitate pro omnibus re petente medicum reperiri.* in parua enim ciuitate appungens aliquis oculos aut incidens ernias nequaquam nutrietur; Roma vero et Alexandria propter multitudinem hominum | sufficientes sunt nutrire et eum, qui quamcumque artem operatur; sed in aliis gentibus

2 aut A: *corr.* B 4 phisiologiam A: *corr.* B 7 adinucem A: *corr.* B 8 partem *edd.*: *corr.* Deichgräber 12 et vocatam] invocatam A: *corr.* B 13 vocatiuam A: *suppl.* Schöne adiderunt A: *corr.* B 15 in *add.* Deichgräber 25 alius aurium et alius] aliarum *edd.*: *sec. versionem Arabicam correximus et supplevimus* 31 repetente A Schöne: repente B

coguntur ciuitates permutare hii tales frequenter †adingeminantes†, ut quod his, qui sunt in Italia, e⟨s⟩t Roma sola, hoc illis fiat verbi gratia Ellada tota.

3. Sed mihi videtur bonum esse, ut adhuc incipiam loqui | de mente
mea. quoniam paruissime particule artis quales sint secundum natu-
ram, iam dictum est, primo nunc apertius determinandum, quas
oportet vocare particulas minimas, exemplum in sermone ponentes
non extra propositum negocium, sed super quidem aliud vtilium debens
esse. sicut ergo corporis nostri particulas | in anothomiis usque ad mini- 2
mas secundum speciem, quas et elementa sensibilia vocamus, conamur
discere, ita oportet et artis minimas particulas. [et elementa sensibilia] 3
organa quidem ut caput, manus, pedes et huiusmodi, horum autem
ipsorum rursus vniuscuiusque sunt partes, velut capitis quidem aures
et facies *et nasus* et collum, | ipsius vero nominati proprie capitis partes
et cerebrum et ambe miringe et craneum et arterie et vene et membrane
et nerui et corium, que omnes secundum primam incisionem inueniun-
tur. harum vero rursus partium singula diuiditur in particulas, et
dictum est de omnibus ipsis in libris De anothomicis tractationibus; in
presenti | vero sufficit proponendo quamcumque ostendere incisionem
corporis usque ad elementa. arteria igitur bitunicalis est secundum 4
sui rationem – monstratum enim est, propter quid tritunicalis et
quadritunicalis apparet –; tunicarum autem eius altera quidem obli-
quos habet inulos, altera vero rectos; ipsos autem inulos in aliam
speciem | non est incidere, sed est indiuisibilis et minima iam hec
particula secundum speciem. igitur et consuetudo est nobis eas quidem, 5
quibus attributus est aliquis unus actus necessarius aut vtilis toti
animali, partes corporis aut organa vocare, minimas vero earum non
particulas solum, sed etiam elementa sensibilia corporis. tales autem
sunt | inoli, qui sunt secundum singulum organorum, sicut sunt arterie
et *vene et nerui* et intestina et venter et matrix et vesica, ex inulis enim
habent *tunicas* consistentes; adhuc autem cum inulis sunt membrane
et colligationes et caro tam simplex quam que est secundum singulum
viscerum propria, quod quidam parenchima seu | co⟨i⟩nfusionem vo-
cant; et cum his est os et cartilago et pinguedo et quodcumque tale

2 et AB: *corr.* Schöne 11 et elementa sensibilia *secl.* Schöne 13 there is what is particularized by this term – that is, "head" *post* quidem *vers. Arab.* 14 et nasus *om. vers. Arab.* 20 sensible *ante* elementa *vers. Arab.* 29 as well as other things that I shall mention later *post* organorum *vers. Arab.* 34 os et] osa A: *corr.* B

†illudque siquidem† sensibilia elementa corporis nostri iuste quis
6 dixerit. altera pars particularum organica erit; non est autem malum
pertransire et hanc: *vene* sunt et *arterie* et nerui et *musculi et tenentes*
et oculi et matrix et intestina et renes et | venter et splen et epar et pulmo
et cor et quecumque alia talia.

4. Secundum igitur similitudinem exempli apunctiuam quidem | suf-
fusionis artem talem partem totius medicatiue oportet putare esse,
qualis est corporis particula quam appellamus organum; singula
aut⟨em⟩ eius particularum proportionalis est sensibilibus corporis
2 elementis. sunt autem partes artis noticie que fiunt in anima nostra,
quas nominant quidam theoremata. prima namque est que | est totius
speciei *organi quod apungitur;* secunda vero particule illius que est
secundum organum, vbi oportet apungere; et tertia que est secundum
commensuritatem dispositionis; et quarta que est circa conuersionem;
et quinta que est a solutione et a motione ipsius suffusionis de loco
quem comprehendit; et sexta que est ex abductione; | et septima que
est de incuneatione – ultime enim sunt hee noticie et minime et simpli-
ces et non habent incisionem ad alias noticias simpliciores eis. noticias
autem vel notiones vel scientias vel theoremata dicere nihil differt ad
3 presens, sicut neque partes et particulas et portiones. scientia igitur
que est de apunctione composita | est ex his que secundum partem
scientiis, quas pertransiui; uniuersa aut⟨em⟩ cura suffusionum indiget
aliquibus aliis noticiis duplicibus secundum genus: prima quidem ordine
4 preparatiua, secunda autem nominata apotherapeutica. si enim
plethoricum sufficienter vel cacochimum vel cephalargicum aliquem
accipiens quis | ducat ad hanc cyrurgiam flegmones aliquos operabitur
tunicarum, que sunt apuncte, et compassionem totius capitis; ut
autem non fiat hoc, preparatiue artis est opus, cuius intentio est absque
superfluitatibus quidem et purum totum corpus, caput aut⟨em⟩ indo-
lorosum ostendere; ex quibus aut⟨em⟩ rursus hoc fiat theorematibus,
elementa artis sunt; | sicut rursus conuenienter, ex quibus post cyrur-
giam absque flegmone quidem oculus sit, innocitum autem totum
caput, et in hoc theoremate elementa medicatiue artis sunt, id est
5 *minime et vltime* particule. hunc ergo sermonem velut exemplum ad
alias vniuersas passiones sciatis esse, et scientiam, que est secundum
singulam earum, | talem esse partem artis, qualis est in animali vocatum

3sq. musculi – intestina *om. vers. Arab.* 9 aut A: *corr.* B 12 que] quod AB: *corr.* Schöne 22 aut A: *corr.* B 29 aut A: *corr.* B 30 aut A: *corr.* B

organum. *adest autem et hoc preter magnum laborem* diligenter deter-
minare totum. sicut enim suffusionis, ita aliquis putabit et flegmonis
simpliciter esse artem curatiuam et similiter ulceris et fracture et
erispile et aliarum passionum. non tamen est ita quod verum. quale | 6
enim est corporis pars quam vocamus organum, talis pars medicatiue 150
est curatiua noticia flegmonis; qualis est particula corporis oculus,
talis pars est scientia curatiua obtalmie – voco autem obtalmiam
flegmonem tunice exterioris ⟨ex⟩ eis que sunt secundum oculum –;
talis etiam est egritudo pulmonis quidem periple⟨u⟩monia, | subcingentis 155
vero costas tunice pleuritis; etenim et hee passiones flegmones quidam
sunt harum particularum. alia quidem ergo est curatiua ars flegmonis,
generaliter intelligere, et alia ⟨eius⟩ que⟨m⟩ determinant cum *patiente*
particula, sicut organum quod generaliter inte⟨l⟩ligitur, aliud est a
determinato organo. quoniam aut⟨em⟩ alia quidem est que fleg|monis, 160
alia vero eius que est in hac particula flegmonis ars curatiua, demon-
stratum est a nobis in Therapeutice methodi scriptionibus.

5. Empericus autem non ait esse aliquam flegmonis ipsius secundum 166
se ipsam generalem curam: sed non est necessarium amplius in talibus
subtilitate verborum vtendo immorari. sed, ut in capitulo dicendo, 2
cum ars medicatiua existat de curis egritudinum, ad primas | et prin- 170
cipalissimas partes diuiduntur notitie cure simplicium egritudinum,
deinde compositarum. quot autem sunt simplices et quot composite
egritudines, ostensum est per vnum librum, qui De differentia egri-
tudinum intitulatur. si vero non solum ab egritudinibus ad sanitatem 3
recuperare est medicatiue, sed etiam sanos in eodem | custodire, sicut 175
in alio a nobis ostensum est libro, pars alia huius [p]artis erit que
vocatur sanatiua, que contradiuiditur dicte scilicet curatiue. huius
autem rursus sunt alie particule theoremata, per que in sanitate
custodietur singula particularum corporis. si vero et tertia aliqua alia 4
est dispositio, quam neutram nominant, necessarium | est et huius 180
prouisiuam esse aliquam aliam partem artis. videtur autem esse talis
dispositio eorum, qui discrasiantur quidem manifeste, non tamen

8 ex *add.* Schöne 9 periplemonia A: *corr.* B 12 eius quem] que *edd.*: *supplevimus* patiente *om. vers. Arab.* 13 inteligitur AB: *corr.* Schöne 14 aut A: *corr.* B 18 However, even following this view, the concept of inflammation cannot be thought of as the same as that of a cataract. For in this latter case the part of the body affected by the ailment now is defined, whereas this was not so in the case of inflammation. *post* curam *vers. Arab.* 26 partis AB: *corr.* Schöne

egrotantium, sed adhuc agere potentium consuetas actiones, vel
nullum habentium in se sensibile malum sed insensibile, sicut est in
185 morsis a cane rabido vel eis, qui sumpserunt deli|terium ab his, que
5 post tempus interficiunt. in huius⟨modi⟩ enim dispositionibus propria
quedam pars artis videtur esse precustoditiua, sicut rursus in his
quidem, qui liberati sunt nuper ab *egritudine*, debiles autem in tantum
existunt adhuc, ut neque balneari possint *neque consueta agere, et*
190 *debilem habent dispositionem corporis*, est | alia particula artis, que
6 vocatur resumptiua. cirocomica vero vocata pars in *nulla* videtur
debere poni dispositione, etenim senectus neque certa est egritudo
7 neque integra sanitas. quidam autem et pedotroficam, id est infantium
educatiuam, nominatam hic locant, dicentes, quod sicut se habet
195 ⟨circa⟩ corpus, ita debet prouidere ars de | neutris dispositionibus.
adhuc autem alii addunt aliam partem, que est circa euexiam, que
vocatur ab aliquibus quidem euectica, ab aliquibus autem *exercitastica*
8 *et ginastica*, ut sint prime et maxime partes artis que est circa corpus:
curatiua, resumptiua, precustoditiua, cirocomica, infantium educatiua,
200 *euectica et sana|tiua*; quibus rursus sic diuisis, sicut ante ostendimus
diuidi curatiua⟨m⟩, ad simplicissimas perueni⟨un⟩t differentias theore-
matum que velut elementa quedam artis ostendimus existere.
207 6. Cuius modi incisio vniuersa secundum dispositionem corporis
facta est. alia vero est que est secundum operationum differentias.
210 quando cyrurgiam et farmaciam et dietam dicunt esse primas | et maxi-
mas medicatiue particulas, fieri videtur aliquibus huius incisio secun-
dum *materiarum differentias*. – omnis enim particula corporis *saluari*
vel iuuari nata est ex dieta vel farmacia vel cyrurgia. – sed magis
proprie dicet quis eas oblata et fientia et que euacuantur et extrorsum
215 2 incidentia. in summa vero dicendo, quicumque a | dispositionibus, quas
ars illa curat et custodit, fecerunt eam que ad partes diuisione⟨m⟩,
totius medicatiue tot particulas dixerunt existere, quot sunt differentie
dispositionum; quidam autem non ab his solum, sed etiam ab omni
vniuersa materia, cuius medicus habet scientiam, qui et phys⟨i⟩olo-
220 gicam et vocatam proprie materialem cum predictis | artis partibus
connumerant. quidam autem ab omnibus operationibus distinguentes

4 huius A: *suppl.* B 7 sq. neque[II] – corporis *om. vers. Arab.* 9 nulla] neutra, *ut ex versione Arabica apparet, recte coni.* Schöne 13 circa *addidimus* neutris] ventris AB: *sec. versionem Arabicam correximus* 19 curatiua AB: *corr.* Schöne peruenit AB: *corr.* Schöne 29 diuisione A: *corr.* B 32 physolog. A: *corr.* B 33 aetiology and *post* et *vers. Arab.*

partes artis vltra dietam et *cyrurgiam et farmaciam* addiderunt signa-
tiuam; quidam autem diuidentes eam in pathognomonicam et pro-
nosticam addiderunt eas cum predictis partibus. plurimi vero emperi- 3
corum, finales partes dicentes esse signatiuam | et curatiuam et vocatam
sanatiuam, in incisione curatiue posuerunt dietam et *farmaciam et
cyrurgiam* vt partes, peccantes quidem in nominationibus – oportet
enim eos non operationum sed scientiarum nomina dicere –, non
tamen in rebus falluntur. melius autem esset, sicut et dicunt quidam 4
ex eis, aliquam quidem partem artis esse | significatiuam, aliam vero
curatiuam, aliam autem sanatiuam; signatiue vero esse partem
pathognomonicam et pronosticam, sicut et curatiue hanc quidem
farmacalem, hanc autem cyrurgicam. precedere igitur ut dicunt pri- 5
mam et generalissimam in partibus medicatiue differentiam in essendo
alias quidem finales, alias vero | constitutiuas, optime dictum est.
finales enim sunt, que finem efficiunt; constitutiue vero, que sunt
constitutionis earum et, ut utique dicat quis, existentie causa. putare 6
tamen signatiuam equiparabilem esse sanatiue et curatiue parti artis
non recte dictum est; de necessitate vero precedit eo, quod non fit
prouidentia alicuius neque cura | absque quod cognoscatur dispositio
circa corpus qualis sit; non tamen ex ipsa significatione peruenitur
ad finem artis. neque etiam similis transitio equiualens est particula
per se inspectioni[s] et hystorie; quare autem, non instat sermo qui
nunc est; sufficienter enim ostensum est per totum vnum librum
per se. et neque | Serapio aliter cognoscebat; sed de hoc quidem ille
cuicumque cura est *eorum que* ⟨*secundum*⟩ *empericam dictionem* per-
transierit hunc librum. ego autem, quia tu eum qui per indicationem
et *methodum* ingressum ad talia nosti, principium sermoni simile
empericis ponens ad continua sermonis transibo.

3 as I said *post* empericorum *vers. Arab.* 12 diet *ante* farmacalem *vers. Arab.* All these parts that we have mentioned you can, if you want, call sciences and you can say that there is here one science relating to cures, another relating to surgery and a third to diet, and the same thing applies to other similar parts of the whole art of medicine. You are not wrong, though, if you talk of "knowledge" or "wisdom" or "theory" in place of "science", as there is no difference between these terms. Nor are you concerned to follow up names but to reach an understanding of the categories involved. *post* cyrurgicam *vers. Arab.* precederunt A: preciderunt B: *corr.* Deichgräber 13 et] in A Schöne: *corr.* B 22 inspectionis AB: *corr.* Schöne 23 by Cassius the theoretician *post* ostensum est *vers. Arab.* 24 the Empiricist *post* Serapio *vers. Arab.* 25 qui A: *corr.* B secundum *addidimus* pertransierunt *edd.*: *correximus*

7. Dico igitur esse medicatiue *primas* quidem et *proprias* et maxime
partes illas, ⟨per⟩ quas nobis aduenit finis artis, alie vero sunt | et hiis
superiores. prime quidem igitur et proxime tot sunt numero, quot sunt
differentie *propriissime* materie eius: propriissima autem materia
medicatiue est dispositione⟨s⟩ nostri corporis, siue due sunt *sicut*
2 *secundum genus* siue tres siue plures. monstratum enim est per unum
librum, qui Ad Trasibulum intitulatur, quoniam duplex | est prima
differentia dispositionum nominata propriis nominibus alte⟨r⟩utra ab
vniuersis hominibus, quarum quidem alteram sanitatem nominare est
nobis consuetudo, alteram vero egritudines. alteriutrius vero rursus
earum species sunt duplices: una quidem est, que est secundum
habitum in utraque dispositione, alia vero secundum | habitudinem.
3 de sanatiua igitur dispositione, que est secundum habitum, procurat
illa pars, quam vocamus sanatiuam, cuius partem precipuam quidam
ponunt *vocatam* euecticam et resumptiuam et cirocomicam. sed in
egritudinibus quidem, que sunt secundum habitum et habitudinem,
non sunt nomina ipsis partibus medicatiue; | harum ipsarum etiam
4 egritudinum alie quidem cronice, alie vero acute nuncupantur. alie
quidem igitur sunt prime et propinquiores artis; alie vero, sine quibus
non sunt he. prima quidem igitur est significatiua; cuius sunt partes
due, hec quidem dignoscitiua presentium, hec vero futurorum pronosticatiua; neque enim absque | quod dignoscatur passio, curam eius est
possibile inuenire, neque absque quod precognoscatur terminus
criseos eius, est possibile curare conueni⟨en⟩t⟨er⟩: has autem rursus
necessarium est precedere illam partem artis, que est circa conditionem
omnium particularum animalis, que in anothomia mortuorum inuenitur; secundario vero | *ex superhabundanti* illam, que est de actibus; et
tertio eam que de utilitate earum est; ipsas aut⟨em⟩ rursus has eam
que de theoria que de elementis corporis, et secundo eam que de
crisibus, et tertio eam que de virtutibus naturalibus, que inveniuntur

2 per *add.* B other parts necessarily precede these *ante* alie *vers. Arab.* 4 propriissime *om. vers. Arab.* materie, *ut ex versione Arabica apparet, recte coni.* Schöne: medicine AB materia *coni.* Schöne: medicina AB 5 dispositione A: *corr.* B 5sq. sicut secundum genus *om. vers. Arab.* 8 alteutra A: *corr.* Schöne 15 vocatam *om. vers. Arab.* as for what deals with health in the second category, this comprises prophylaxis *post* euecticam *vers. Arab.* 24 or what shape the disease will take *post* eius *vers. Arab.* conuenit A: *corr.* B 27 ex superhabundanti *om. vers. Arab.* 28 aut A: *corr.* B 30 crisibus *ex* crasibus *vel* κρισ. *ex* κρασ. *corruptum est* and spiritual *post* naturalibus *vers. Arab.*

cum anothomia que in animalibus; ad tot enim principia resoluitur
pars signi|ficatiua, quam precedere curatiuam et sanatiuam penitus 285
dicimus. ostensa sunt autem omnia illa in propriis tractatibus. est 5
tamen alia pars artis, quam adiungunt significatiue, precedens cura-
tiuam, que pars est de notione omnium causarum egrotatiuarum et
sanatiuarum, quam materialem quidam nuncupant, existens cognos-
citiua | omnium causarum. *maxime* vero causarum in eis que offeruntur 290
et que fiunt et euacuantur et extrorsum incidunt considerantur, con-
siderando videlicet virtutem vniuscuiusque predictorum. quam
aut⟨em⟩ vtilitatem arti prebent hec, per Terapeuticam methodum
ostensum est.

8. Que quidem igitur ⟨secundum⟩ propriissimam materiam medi- 298
catiue inventio partium eius, ex tali; que vero est secundum secundo |
propriam, sic: corpus hominis medicatiue artis est materia secunda 300
et, ⟨ut⟩ utique dicat quis, secundum accidens eo, quod huius dispo-
sitiones sunt sanitas et egritudo. est enim et phisice sermo, tamen 2
et secundum accidens, corpus eo, quod est generabile et corruptibile.
naturalis vero phylosophia de eis, que sunt in generatione et cor|rup- 305
tione, considerat, et propter hoc primo et huic scientie est materia
generatio et propter hanc generabile corpus. iccirco enim et humanum
corpus est materia naturalis, eo quod est generabile et cor-
ruptibile; medicatiue vero non propter hoc, sed in quantum est
passibile et *sanabile*. quia igitur materia quodammodo est medicatiue | 3
corpus hominis, tot ostendet incisiones hec ars secundum partem, 310
quot et corpus; due vero erunt eorum differentie secundum genus,
altera quidem circa elementales particulas, altera vero circa organicas.
†*pars aut rursus indiuisibilis numero. particule animalis aut sunt*
tam elementales quam organice†, et harum rursus vniuscuiusque | una- 315
queque passio erit propria pars artis, quam ostendimus ad actus qui
secundum partem diuidi[tur] in sermone de apunctione; harum enim
scientie sunt elementales particule totius artis. in eis vero que sunt
secundum farmaciam, sunt ille, que sunt de simplicibus farmaciis
vniuscuiusque, sicut in eis, que secundum dietam, ille | que sunt simpli- 320

7 causarum[II]] material causes *vers. Arab.* 10 aut A: *corr.* B 12 secundum *add.* B 15 ut *add.* Schöne 20 accidentally *ante* generabile *vers. Arab.* 25 differentie] prime types *vers. Arab.* 27sq. pars – organice] When we divide these with all their subdivisions, the number of the sections of medicine will be that of these two classes of parts with the ailments that can affect each of them added in. *vers. Arab.* 30 diuiditur AB: *corr.* Schöne

4 cium dietematum. non solum autem ex huius materie incisio⟨ne⟩ usque
ad ultimas et elementales artis particulas accedit, sed etiam ex ea,
que parum ante dicta est. adhuc autem secundum alium modum fit
5 diuisio. fer[e] enim nos velle diuidere vsque ad vltimas particulas,
325 vnum genus dispositionum que secundum egri | tudines proponentibus
nobis. erit igitur in hoc prima quidem incisio, quod hee quidem omiomeris, hee vero organicis accidunt, sicut in libro De differentia egritudinum ostensum est; secunda vero, quod alie quidem ipsarum sunt
simplices, alie vero composite, sicut et hoc in illo libro ostensum est.
330 6 necessarium igitur est curatiuam | scientiam minimas et elementales
habere particulas easdem his que antea dicte sunt. fer[e] enim, si ita contingat, calidam egritudinem velle nos curare: minime primo quidem ⟨in⟩ curam eius cognoscere est necessarium, quoniam quidem contraria contrariorum sunt sanationes – hoc enim ostensum est esse
335 commune et primum omnium –; | deinde quoniam id, quod est in primo
gradu calidum, ei quod est secundum primum gradum frigidum; deinde consequenter gradus calidarum egritudinum et farmacorum
7 infrigidantium, sicut in libris qui de farmaciis ostensum est. quo et
manifestum, quoniam, vndecunque inceperit quis incidere, si recte
340 incidit usque ad vltima | et elementalia theoremata pe⟨r⟩uenit ad
scientiam eorum, que dicta sunt.

346 9. Vt autem clarius adhuc sciatis, hic alicuius alterius incisionis
faciam memoriam et maxime eius qua multotiens usus fui. eorum enim, que sunt circa corpus hominis, alia quidem sunt secundum
350 naturam, alia vero preter naturam; et eorum, que preter | naturam,
alia quidem [secundum] egritudines, alia vero sinthomata horum, ⟨alia⟩ autem cause. eorum quidem, que sunt secundum naturam, scientiam custodie oportet habere medicum, eorum vero, que preter naturam, interemptionis *communis*. quale autem esse convenit vtrum-
355 2 que, ostensum est per alia. sed ad presens id, quod proponitur, | exami-
nandum est; singulum predictorum oportet diuidere propria incisione; *seorsum* autem de uno quoque scriptum est, de egritudinibus quidem in libro De differentia egritudinum, de causis vero seorsum in alio libro,
3 sicut et de sinthomatibus in alio. et sanorum etiam differentias osten-

1 incisio AB: *corr.* Schöne 4 fere A: *corr.* B 11 fere A: *corr.* B 13 in *add.* Schöne 20 peuenit A: *corr.* B 26 secundum *secl.* Schöne 27 alia *sec. versionem Arabicam addidimus* quidem *post* eorum *transposuimus, post* sunt *edd.* 29 communis *om. vers. Arab.* but this is not the place to mention *ante* quale *vers. Arab.* 32 seorsum *om. vers. Arab.*

dimus per Sanatiuam operam, in qua et, | quomodo oportet de unaquaque earum providere, scriptum est, *facta resolutione* egritudinum et causarum et sinthomatum in Terapeutica.

Et namque secundum huius⟨modi⟩ incisionem ea, que sunt prima et 4 principalissima artis, non alia a dictis superius inuenientur esse. similiter autem et ea que secundario sunt propria et tertio, sicut antea| dictum est et quoniam hec ipsa oportet incidere et, si recte incidantur, necesse est incisionem desinere usque ad elementarissimas scientias. quoniam autem multiformiter adest incidere singulum eorum, que 5 proposita sunt, dictum est non solum simpliciter, sed a dyale⟨c⟩ticissimis phylosophorum ac etiam per exempla a Platone | per duos libros, scilicet per Sophisten et Politicum.

Non igitur turbet te multitudo incisionum, neque si secundum 6 diuersos modos inciserunt medicatiuam anteriores, sed si nihil eorum, que occurrunt, obmissum est, considera; quicumque enim hec obseruat, moderate diuidit. optimum est autem, sicut prius dictum est, prin-| cipium facere a [p]propriissima materia, et deinde alia secundum prius dictam methodum ad[d]icere.

2 facta resolutione] and I analysed the problem until I arrived at the simple and elementary sciences. I did the same *vers. Arab.* 4 huius AB: *suppl.* Schöne 7 until one reaches what is simple and ultimate *post* incidere *vers. Arab.* 10 dyaleticiss. A: *corr.* B 12 Sophisticum *edd.*: *correximus* 17 ppropr. A: *corr.* B 18 addicere A: *corr.* B

GALIENI

DE CAVSIS CONTENTIVIS

CONSPECTVS SIGLORVM

P = Parisinus lat. 6865, s. XIV, f. 5^r–6^v
D = Dresdensis Db 93, s. XV, f. 443^r–445^r

GALIENI

DE CAVSIS CONTENTIVIS

1. Stoycos philosophos noui primos contentiuam causam que et 6 Kalbfleisch
coniuncta dicitur nominare. volunt enim ex quatuor quidem elementis
facta esse uocata ab Aristotile quidem omiomera corpora, primo-
genita autem a Platone, ex hiis autem alia corpora | componi. elemen- 2 7
torum autem quedam quidem materialia nuncupant, quedam autem
actiua et uirtuosa, et contineri dicunt a uirtuosis materialia, et esse
ignem quidem et aërem actiua, terram uero et aquam materialia, et
pertransire tota per tota in concrecionibus, scilicet uirtuosa per mate-
rialia, ut aërem et ignem per aquam et terram, et esse aërem quidem
frigidum, ignem uero calidum, et congregari et impilari substantiam
ab aërea natura, extendi uero et effundi et multum accipere locum ab
ignea et esse leptomerea quidem elementa actiua, grossiparcia uero
reliqua. spiritum autem uocant leptomeream substantiam omnem, 3
et eius opus esse continere alia corpora physica et ea que animalium.
nomino autem physica, quorum generatio non ab hominibus sed a
natura fit: talia autem sunt es et *ferrum* et aurum et ligna et parti-
cularum que in animalibus prime et omiomere uocate, scilicet neruus
et uena et arteria et cartillago et os et quecumque alie tales. sicut 4
autem homines ligna per collam et colligationem et clauos et lutum et
gipsum et calcem couniunt ad inuicem, sic uidemus et naturam per
colligationem ⟨*et*⟩ *cartillaginem et carnem* vnientem et applicantem ad
inuicem omnes particulas animalis. et uocare licet ei quicumque 5
uoluerit coniunctas causas compositarum particularum eas que
†*naturam*† operantur simplicium que sunt in eis, sicut in exterioribus
quecumque non natura sed ars humana compaginat scilicet lutum et
gipsum et calcem et quecumque alia talia hiis utilitatibus famulantur.

9 dynamic and *ante* actiua *vers. Arab.* 23 et[I] *addidimus* 26 naturam] union *vers. Arab.*

8 vocantur autem a Stoycis non hec | coniuncte cause *entium*, sed
suptilipartis substantia materialis.

2. Athineum igitur Attaleum, qui spiritualem nominatam here-
sim in medicatiua primo cepit, coniunctam uocare causam egritudinum
decens est ceu a Stoicorum heresi deductum (conuersatus enim fuit
cum Posidonio), alios uero medicos, quicumque dogmata colunt alia,
coniunctam causam singule egritudinum non congruit querere, sicut
neque omiomerorum corporum que secundum naturam habent: ergo
neque differentias causarum sicut Athineus dicebat tres esse primas
2 et generalissimas contingit dicere eos. differentie uero, quas dicebat
Athineus esse tres, sunt hee: prima quidem coniunctarum, secunda
9 uero antecedentium, | tercia autem in procatarticarum materia con-
3 tinetur. vocant autem ita omnia quecumque extra corpus existentia
nocent ei operantia egritudinem; de genere autem operantium intus
existencia antecedentes cause vocantur; alterationes autem innati
spiritus que fiunt ab hiis et etiam ab extrinsecis humectato et siccato
et *infrigidato et calefacto corpore* coniunctas egritudinum ait esse causas,
pertransit enim spiritus iste per omiomera corpora sibi ipsi coalterans
4 ea. multociens igitur confestim a procatarticis causis fieri dicunt
coniunctas: quando enim perustus quis fuerit a sole, transmutari aiunt
necessario nostrum innatum spiritum et fieri calidiorem se ipso, infrigi-
dato autem a frigore alterari secundum frigiditatem; paruis autem
hiis fientibus nondum egrotare nos, si uero in tantum euertatur a
crasi que secundum naturam particula, ut iam noceatur actus eius,
egritudinem esse eius secundum discrasiam factam, causam coniunc-
tam habentem spiritum calefactum immoderate uel infrigidatum uel
5 siccatum ⟨uel humectatum⟩. antecedentes uero egritudinum causas
nominant qui ab hac heresi et eos qui in corpore generantur humores,
quando immoderatius fuerint calidi et frigidi et *sicci et humidi;* disponi
enim ab eis in tempore solida corpora et propterea et actus eorum
10 6 noceri. huius generis esse | putant et ferarum uenena, quale est et
rabidi canis et omnia mortalia et deliteria uocata farmaca, licet que-
dam horum nullum manifestum malum faciant in animalium cor-
poribus eo quod in multo tempore paulatim faciant alterationem et
non repente. ac etiam sanguinis multitudinem aliquando egritudinum
causam fieri dicunt.

1 entium *om. vers. Arab.* 17 corpore *om. vers. Arab.* 21 necessario *om. vers. Arab.* 27 uel humectatum, *ut ex versione Arabica apparet, recte add.* Kalbfleisch

3. Ego autem quoniam quidem ex igne et *aqua et aëre et terra* est
generatio naturalibus corporibus, ab Ypocrate primo omnium mon-
stratum esse extimo, et differre nichil, si aliquis sic sicut ego nunc
nominibus utatur secundum substantiam nominans elementa ignem
et aquam et aërem et terram uel secundum qualitates *calidum et frigi-
dum et siccum et humidum;* non tamen extimo spiritum prius in *ani-
malibus uel* naturalibus corporibus alteratum sibi ipsi coalterare reli-
qua. non enim permanet talis spiritus qualis a principio erat, quando 2
concretio eius que ad alia fiebat: cum enim comisceantur quatuor
elementa per tota, aliud unum quoddam fit corpus quintum ex qua-
tuor, aliud existens ab eorum singulo, sicut in tetrafarmaca uocata
uirtute. permixtis enim ad inuicem per totum cera et *resina et pice* et 3
adipe nullum illorum adhuc | manet tale quale ante erat, sed unum 11
aliud corpus quintum, aliud quam singulum illorum quatuor fit, eo
quod nullum sincerum adhuc secundum sui ipsius naturam in concre-
tione saluatur, sicut in solidorum corporum mixtione. si enim quam 4
maxime terens certitudinaliter ut puluerosa facias *spumam argenti*
et uitreolum et eruginem eris et cerusam permiscueris adinuicem,
singulum *adhuc* manet tale quale a principio erat.

4. Quocirca quando aliqua extrinsecarum causarum alterationem
aliquam in omiomeris operatur corporibus, calefaciens uel infrigidans
uel siccans uel humectans, tocius compositi transmutationem facit,
prius autem rationabile est alterari humida corpora, sicut apparet et
in exterioribus, quando similiter patiuntur solari caliditate aqua et
lapis; adhuc autem cicius quam aqua alterari natus est aër. ita denique 2
et ego multociens in meis submemorationibus dixi uirtutem *causarum*
extrinsecarum alterare primo quidem aëream et spiritualem nomina-
tam substantiam, secundo uero eam que humorum, deinde sic ad eam
que solidorum accedere et huius quidem primo quidem ad pinguedinem
et carnem, secundo autem ad *omnia* membranosa et neruosa corpora,
deinde ad cartillagines et ossa. continetur enim in spaciositatibus 3
corporis sicut humiditas ita et | aërea substantia, eum autem qui in 12
solidis particulis spiritum prius quam humores non utique dicet aliquis
alterari, eo quod non permanet is spiritus; si autem permaneret, 4
alteraretur utique cito *secundum se ipsum.* denique paratissime sus-

6sq. animalibus uel *om. vers. Arab.* 19 adhuc *om. vers. Arab.* 26 causarum *om. vers. Arab.* 30 omnia *om. vers. Arab.* 35 secundum se ipsum *om. vers. Arab.*

cipit eam que est ex calefacientibus et infrigidantibus et humectantibus
et siccantibus alterationem, sicut licet euidenter uidere in continente
nos aëre: prius enim rationabile est alterari leptomerea, et hoc idem
5 opinati sunt qui ab Athineo. uidemus enim manifeste a solari calidi-
tate in caumatibus que sub cane primo quidem aërem calefieri, parum
uero post aquam, si aqua fuerit quod comprehenditur uel aliud humi-
dum, postea uero solida corpora; ac etiam in eo quod non adhuc a sole
calefiunt occidente eo primo quidem aër ad eam que a principio redit
6 crasim, consequenter autem aqua, postremo uero lapides. quod enim
est facile alterabile, citiores facit eas que ad alterutra transmutationes
quam quod est difficile alterabile; quod autem tempore multo eam que
ad id quod preter naturam euersionem habet, hoc et reditum qui ad id
7 quod secundum naturam habet tardum. sicut igitur in inanimatis
corporibus, sic et in animalibus aërea quidem substantia citissimam
suscipit transmutationem, humida uero tardiorem, solida uero omnium
8 tardissimam. quocirca cum estuatio uel infrigidatio in aliqua particula
fit, primo quidem in ea aërea natura alteratur contenta in intermediis
18 solidorum cor|porum spaciositatibus et secundum multas que in
ipsis concauitates, consequenter autem humida substantia, deinde ea
que solidorum, que et particule nostri corporis sunt.

5. Si tamen intellexeris totas per totum concretas esse tres substan-
tias, non adhuc competit dicere primo quidem alterari aëream,
2 secundo uero humidam et terciam ultra hanc terream. hoc enim, scili-
cet per tota permisceri iddem est huic, scilicet totaliter alterari mix-
torum singulum, quoniam, si quale erat ante adhuc nunc permanet,
iuxtapositio eorum erit secundum paruas partes et non per tota con-
3 cretio. sed hoc quidem Empedocles uolebat, mixtione quatuor ele-
mentorum et non concretione naturalia corpora consistere putans, et
secundum hoc communicat hoc suum dogma hiis qui circa Epicurum
et Democritum; non tamen Stoyci philosophi iuxtapositionem esse
4 putant, sicut neque Aristotiles neque spirituales medicorum. hec
quidem *ex superhabundanti* dixi repugnantiam ostendentia ad inuicem
dictorum a Stoycis; non enim concordant ad inuicem hoc, scilicet
per tota concerni elementa et hoc, scilicet primum in eis alterari spiri-
tum; et absque hiis autem concludi potest id quod est utile medicis.
14 5 siue | enim totam dicamus simul alterari patientem particulam siue
prius quidem spiritum, per medium autem ipsum alia, curam neces-
sarium est eandem facere, eis quidem que infrigidata sunt corporibus
offerendo calefacientia, eis vero que calefacta immoderate infrigidan-

tia, sicut et eis que siccata humectantia, eis autem que humectata siccantia.

6. Quicumque autem aiunt inutilem esse medicis elementorum
cognitionem uel utilem quidem, aliam uero aliquam ⟨quam⟩ Stoycam
amplectuntur, hiis *possibile* est supponere contentiuam causam vnius-
cuiusque entium esse, et a multis est audire dicentibus ceu ⟨*in*⟩*demon-* 2
strabile⟨*m*⟩ *et a se ipso credibilem* dignitatem hoc, scilicet non posse
ullum corpus habitum habentium absque continente causa esse. aiunt
autem non in omnibus corporibus contentiuam uirtutem existere,
sed in solis hiis que difficile solubilem et difficile sparsibilem habent
substantiam; talia autem esse corpora adamantem et lapides et
ostraca et ferrum et quecumque talia. interimit autem ratio eorum se 3
ipsam: si enim singulum entium causa indiget contentiua, qua sine
non est possibile existere omnino, utique et causam illam vnum aliquod
entium existentem ab alia causa necessarium est contineri | et illam 15
rursus ab alia et hoc in infinitum extendi nusquam stare potens. si 4
uero quedam quidem entium se ipsa continere dixerint, quedam autem
aliis indigere, quod quidem facile sparsibilem habet substantiam,
rationabile erit continente ipsum indigere, quod autem constrictam et
contentam diligenter, nullo indigere tali, et propter hoc homines et
ligna et lapides et argentum et aurum et ferrum et es et quecumque
alia talia absque continere debentibus ea *esse*, aquam uero et vinum et
acetum et mel in lagenis et doliis immittere, cum se ipsa continere
nequeant. ergo non est decens alio indigere solidum corpus continere 5
debente id, propterea quod hoc sic est durum et solidum, quoniam
continere se ipsum natum est. hoc autem et Stoycorum tangit
opinionem, quando aliquod corpus terreum quale est adamas et lapis
contineri dicunt a spirituali substantia: facile sparsibilem autem
uidemus naturam spiritus, difficile solubilem uero eam que terre, et
cum hoc nec excogitari potest quod *terream* aliquam substantiam, etsi
minima secundum magnitudinem fuerit sicut athomi qui sunt secun-
dum Epicurum, *continere eam*. aut enim non est omnino existencia 6
elementi terrei nec minimis terre partium absque spirituali substantia
existere queuntibus, aut si sunt alique partes et minime particule terre
ipse secundum se ipsas absque quod coaceruentur spiritu omnino,

4 quam *add.* Kalbfleisch 6 indemonstrabilem, *ut ex versione Arabica apparet, recte corr.* Kalbfleisch 22 debentium P: debiliter D: debentibus *coni.* Kalbfleisch esse] *ΕΙΝΑΙ ex ΘΕΙΝΑΙ corruptum esse videtur* 30 terream *om. vers. Arab.*

utique hee continere se ipsas nate sunt. sed hoc quidem sicut et aliud quid antedictorum *ex superhabundanti* dicatur. |

16 7. Mirari autem adest de medicis quicumque cognitione elementorum non indigere medicatiuam dicentes causas nominant contentiuas: nullum enim entium ut contineatur videtur indigere alia substantia,
2 sed est unumquodque sibi sufficiens ad esse. periclitatur igitur si aliquis diligenter considerat omnem causam non substantie alicuius *primo* sed generationis existere causam, non autem principium eius que fit substantie: generatio enim uelut uia est ad substantiam ducens, et propterea *spiritus* est solummodo causa generationis, quicquid
3 autem est ingenitum non habet causam. propterea et Plato dicebat in Tymeo: „omne quod fit a causa aliqua necessario fit, omnino enim est impossibile absque causa generationem habere"; sed quod iam factum est, a causa quidem aliqua necessarium est fore factum, nunc autem non adhuc indiget causa.

8. Vnde autem decepti quidam contentiuam causam vniuscuiusque entium esse dicunt? michi quidem videtur ex eo quod non distingunt
17 que simpliciter et proprie esse dicuntur et | que non *simpliciter neque*
2 *proprie* sed cum adiectione. quorum enim non permanent particule, hec nec simpliciter sunt entia, sicut uox et ambulatio et omnis actio et passio et vno sermone motus siue secundum lationem siue secundum alterationem fiat: horum enim *omnium* uidebuntur esse alique cause contentiue iis qui non diligenter considerant naturam eorum, que in fieri acquirunt esse non simpliciter existens, quoniam neque permanet
3 eorum pars sicut entium vniuscuiusque. tale quid enim et in pulsibus accidit: quoniam enim uident in omni tempore uite secundum arterias et cor incessanter fieri, esse eos extimant, et nimirum non *simpliciter* existentibus ipsis sicut arterie et cor et alie particule corporis nostri: in fieri enim inest pulsibus esse nulla ipsorum parte permanente; putant autem quidam permanere particulas, non potentes distinguere
4 quod fit ab ente. quod fit denique simile est fluentibus aquis, quod uero est permanentibus: sic namque et in fluminibus et maxime quando aliquis *subito* ea aspicit putat permansibilem esse eorum substantiam, et nimirum nulla parte eorum permanente, sed quia communis species semper permanet fluentis aque, ad fantasiam uenimus multotiens non
5 fluere sed permanere ipsa. ita autem et pulsuum qui quidem iam factus est, non est, sicut neque qui futurus est; solus autem qui subincidit

18sq. simpliciter neque proprie *om. vers. Arab.* 22 omnium *om. vers. Arab.* 27 simpliciter *om. vers. Arab.*

digitis, est, non autem simpliciter et iste, sed in fieri acquirens esse:
nulla igitur permanet | particula eius, corruptis mox simul omnibus 18
cum ipso *fieri*; forsan autem infallacius est *non simul cum ipso fieri*
dicere, sed simul cum *facto esse*. causas autem generationis eius tres 6
ostendimus esse, scilicet utilitatem, cuius gratia fit, et uitalem uirtu-
tem, a qua fit, et corpus arterie et cordis, quod organum eius est: si
igitur uoluerit quis eas contentiuas causas nominare generationis
pulsuum, sicut et ego multociens nominaui in opera que De pulsibus
non proprie quidem sed abusiue gratia manifeste simul et compendiose
doctrine, non male utetur nuncupatione. talis causa est et plumbum in 7
aliquibus statuis, quecumque inclinationem habentes ad id quod ante
caderent utique, nisi in subiectis lapidibus ⟨pedibus⟩ earum detentis
manerent in statione per ligaturam | que per plumbum, inclinatione 19
earum quantum in propria natura adhuc durante, prohibita uero eo
quod optinentur et trahuntur uersus retro per plumbum. quocirca et 8
hic alicuius fientis et non entis simpliciter est plumbum causa, sed
propterea quod hoc fit omni tempore et manet sibi ipsi simile, fanthasia
fit videntibus ceu una *athoma* re; est autem neque *athoma* neque
omnino *substantia* aliqua, sed generatio in materiis *athomis* multis
vnius *speciei*. quale quid et hiis qui spasmantur inest: manente enim 9
ea que operatur hoc symptoma dispositione spasmus quidem est id
quod fit, causa uero que manet contentiua generationis eius. eodem 10
autem modo uigilationis desipientie *scotomie* tussis disnie amblyopie
et difficultatis auditus cause quedam sunt in corpore predictarum
passionum factiue; vocant autem quidam ipsas dispositiones *passiones*
seu egritudines et harum dispositionum simptoma aiunt esse nocu-
menta actuum, causas uero ipsarum dispositiones corporum. quoniam 11
igitur rationem cause habent dispositiones respectu nocumentorum,
confitentur omnes, sicut et quoniam auxiliorum prima intentio dis-
positiones sunt; sed ambiguitas facta est de ipsa nuncupatione. tamen 12
sequens est primis quidem quicumque dispositiones corporum nomi-
nant egritudines, | nullam esse causam dicere contentiuam egritudi- 20
num, aliis autem id quod parum ante dixi, scilicet ex abusione inferre
nomen contentiuarum causarum dispositionibus, ceu nocumento
actuum ab eis fiente.

3 non simul cum ipso fieri *om. vers. Arab.* 6 eorum *codd.*: *sec. versionem Arabicam correximus* 12 pedibus, *ut ex versione Arabica apparet, recte add.* Kalbfleisch 23 scotomie] stupor *vers. Arab.* 25sq. passiones seu *om. vers. Arab.* 27 others call the types of functional injury diseases *post* actuum *vers. Arab.*

9. In egrotantibus igitur sermo qui de contentiuis causis ut figuraliter
dicatur talis quidem est, in sanis autem corporibus sicut ante dixi, si
quidem omiomera fuerint, nullam habentibus nobis dicere causam
contentiuam, si uero organa et composita, habentibus dicere ea que
adapplicant et copulant primorum et simplicium *corporum* substan-
2 tias. Stoycus uero, sicut dixi, et ipsa prima corpora omiomera con-
tentiuam causam habere dixit, scilicet spiritus substantiam; sed
secunda et composita corpora, sicut et ante dixi, similiter artificialibus
corporibus ab aliquibus causis contineri omnibus confiteri necessarium
3 est et non solum Stoycis. sicut enim in *tubis* et lectis et *cauernis* et
nauibus et domibus compositionem eorum operantur mansiuam lutum
et gipsum et calx et clauus et quecumque alia hiis similia, secundum
eandem rationem in corporibus sunt colligationes et tenontes et carnes
et cartillagines; ossium uero quedam et absque hiis ad difficile solu-
bilem perueniunt coagulationem, sicut et quedam secundum coappli-
cationem, uel clauationem uel suturam uel armoniam apparent com-
4 posita. tales autem quasdam dicent esse compositiones et ipsorum
21 omiomerorum et | *per se prodeuntium* corporum, quicumque elementa
ponunt ea que anarma ab Asclipiade vocantur et que ab aliis minima
5 et ⟨ab eis qui⟩ Epicuri atomi. ex quali enim complicatione eorum
concreta esse aiunt naturalia corpora, ipsis quidem primis et simpli-
cibus, que utique et elementa sensibilium sunt, nullam habentibus
contentiuam causam, quecumque uero ex eis componuntur, compo-
6 sitionem ipsam habere potentibus pro causa. contentiuam igitur aiunt
causam estuationis factam in capite caliditatem, ulceris uero diui-
sionem, non conspicientes quoniam eandem rem per alia uocabula
exponunt: nichil enim aliud est estuatio quam facta in capite caliditas
a solaribus radiis, sicut neque ulcus aliquid aliud quam carnis diuisio.
7 hec autem vox, scilicet diuisio, generalem rem quandam indicat
fientem in omnibus continuis corporibus, solutionem enim continuita-
tis que in hiis fit diuisionem nominamus; ulcus autem et fractura et
scissio et uulsio duarum rerum intellectum comprehendit, scilicet
ipsius diuisionis et corporis in quo fit: secundum cutim namque
diuisione fiente, sicut et secundum subiectam ei carnem vlcus nomi-
22 natur passio, secundum musculum uero scissio, osse autem | patiente
fracturam nominamus egritudinem, sicut et uulsionem neruosa parti-
cula diuulsa.

5 corporum *om. vers. Arab.* 12 pegs, wedges *post* clauus *vers. Arab.*
18 per se prodeuntium *om. vers. Arab.* 20 ab eis qui *addidimus*

10. Igitur in hiis talibus quidem dispositiones corporum sunt mani-
feste, pleuresis autem et peripleumonie et lienterie et litargie et frenesis
dispositiones quidem sunt immanifeste, *passiones* uero que ab eis fiunt
manifeste, scilicet desipientie et uigilie et dolores et disnie et tusses et
excreationes preter naturam et *quecumque alia hiis similia* uidentur
concidere egrotantibus. quorum si quis dicat esse causas contentiuas 2
generationis dispositiones corporum, infallacius dicet quam omnino
dicendo simpliciter eorum esse causas contentiuas dispositiones absque
quod adiciat hoc, scilicet generationis. huius igitur dicet utique quis 3
rationabiliter dispositiones causas contentiuas, ipsorum autem sympto-
matum que fiunt nequaquam, nisi abutens quis ut dixi nominare uo-
luerit ita. igitur empericis quidem sequens est ea que per sensus ad 4
noticiam ueniunt eorum que accidunt nobis cum egrotamus passiones
et simptomata uocare, quecumque uero ipsorum uisa sunt multociens
ad inuicem primam generationem habere et consequenter augmentum
statumque et declinationem nominare egritudines et passiones et
concursus; uolunt enim concursus nomen significatiuum existere |
aceruationis alicuius fientium simul et augmentum et solutionem 23
suscipientium symptomatum. nominare autem consueuerunt hec talia 5
symptomata et signa: et namque uere sunt signa constructionum non
apparentium quas causas nominant illarum *passionum* que apparent;
non tamen extimant secundum ueritatem signari dispositiones ex eis,
quoniam neque concedunt omnino eam que ex indicatiuis signis
noticiam, quam nescio qualiter assueuerunt omnes iam nominare
cathalipsim, id est comprehensionem. neque enim ratio ista *que sub-* 6
infertur, cuius altera quidem sumptionum est talis „si hec sunt signa,
hee sunt cause", secunda uero „si hee sunt cause, hec est cura", sunt
de hiis que placent empericis, sed ut confessas dogmaticis medicis eas
sumentes *ceu consequens inferunt coattractionem causarum*. inter dog- 7
maticos uero ipsos disceptatio | nichil conferens ad medicinalia opera 24
adinuicem facta est, aliis quidem ut dixi dispositiones extimantibus
esse egritudines, aliis autem sequentia eas nocumenta actuum. sed 8
cum confessum sit ab utrisque a dispositionibus inueniri indicatiue
curam, facile notum est quod logica sit disceptatio, neque conferens
neque nocens nobis ad artis opera: etenim qui eas egritudines uocat
consimiliter ei qui causas egritudinum nominat indicationem cure ab
illis accipit et *auxilia quibus eas destruit assumit*.

5 quecumque alia hiis similia *om. vers. Arab.*

INDEXES

PROPER NAMES

Arabic-Greek

فى الأسباب (scil. فى أسباب الأمراض) *Περὶ τῶν ἐν τοῖς νοσήμασιν αἰτίων* 48,7

فى أصناف الأمراض *Περὶ διαφορᾶς νοσημάτων* 36,8 46,11 48,6sq.

فى الأعراض *Περὶ τῆς τῶν συμπτωμάτων διαφορᾶς vel Περὶ αἰτίων συμπτωμάτων* 48,8

علاج التشريح *Περὶ ἀνατομικῶν ἐγχειρήσεων* 30,9

فى النبض *Περὶ σφυγμῶν* 66,7

حنين بن إسحق 26,5.18 30,2.3 32,11.13 34,11.15 62,23

دكسبس ، دكسفس *Δέξιππος* 86,10 106,1.4

ديمقريطس *Δημόκριτος* 60,4

الرجل الذى ظنّ بابقراط أنّه كان يغذو المريض فى كلّ يوم ، هذا الطبيب العجيب ، المتطبّب ، صاحبك هذا *et sim.* 80,13.14 84,17sq. 86,15 98,10sq. 100,4sq. 7 102,5sq. 106,10

رومية *Ῥώμη* 26,22 28,13.17

سارافس من أصحاب التجربة *Σεραπίων ὁ ἐμπειρικός* 40,27

القدماء من شعراء اليونانيّين 108,3.11

شيعة ← ابيقورس

صاحبك هذا ← الرجل الذى . . .

أصحاب التجربة (التجارب) *οἱ ἐμπειρικοί* 26,9.16.18.19.20sq. 34,26 40,2. 27 42,3 70,19 72,5

أصحاب الرأى *οἱ δογματικοί* 26,16. 19.20

أصحاب الروح *οἱ πνευματικοί* 54,4 → طبيب

أصحاب المظلّة *οἱ Στωϊκοί* 52,2 54,1.5 60,4.6.16 62,10 68,7sq. 9sq.

أصحاب القياس *οἱ δογματικοί* 72,5.6

أصحاب النحو من اليونانيّين *οἱ γραμματικοί* 104,2

طبيب ← الرجل الذى . . .

الأطبّاء 54,6 76,13 82,7 86,11 108,2

أهل دهرنا من الأطبّاء 82,9 90,12 106,14

من عزّ قبله (بقراط) من الأطبّاء 94,2

من يقول بالروح من الأطبّاء *οἱ πνευματικοί* 60,5

المتطبّب ← الرجل الذى . . .

فانطس *Φαῶν* 108,6.10

الفلاسفة *οἱ φιλόσοφοι* 48,18 52,2 60,4

فلاطن ، افلاطن *Πλάτων* 52,4

سوفسطيس *Σοφιστής* 48,20

طيماوس *Τίμαιος* 64,1

فوليطيقوس *Πολιτικός* 48,21

فيلسطيون ، فيليسطيون *Φιλιστίων* 108,5. 10

فولبس *Πόλυβος* 108,13

القدماء → شعراء *οἱ παλαιοί* 24,3

قسيس النظّار *Κάσσιος ὁ σκεπτικός* 40,26

أهل قنيدس *Κνίδιος* 100,1

بلاد الهند *Ἰνδία* 108,9

اليونانيّون ← شعراء ، أصحاب النحو 34,12 62,24

بلد اليونانيّين *Ἑλλάς* 28,18

English

Arabic

Latin (for De Partibus Artis Medicativae and De Causis Contentivis)

English (for De Diaeta in Morbis Acutis secundum Hippocratem)

LIST OF SPECIAL TERMS IN GREEK-LATIN-ENGLISH-ARABIC

ἀγμός, κάταγμα	fractura	fracture	كسر
ἀγρυπνία	vigilatio, vigilia	insomnia	سهر
ἀδάμας	adamas	adamant	حجر إلصنام
αδιαίρετος	indivisibilis	indivisible	لا يحتمل القسمة
αἷμα	sanguis	blood	دم
αἴσθησις	sensus	sense	حس
τἰσθητός	sensibilis	sensible	محسوس
ἀὸ αἰτιολογικόν (μέρος)	causiologica (pars)	aetiology	الكلام فى الأسباب
αἴτιον, αἰτία	causa	cause	سبب
αἴτιον προηγούμενον	causa antecedens	prior cause	سبب سابق
αἴτιον προκαταρκτικόν	causa procatartica	immediate cause	سبب بادئ
αἴτιον συνεκτικόν	causa contentiva, c. coniuncta	cohesive cause	سبب ماسك
ἀμβλυωπία	amblyopia	dulled eyesight	ظلمة البصر
τὸ ἀναληπτικόν (μέρος)	resumptiva (pars)	the recuperative section	تلاف ، تلافى الصحّة
ἄναρμος	anarmus	disunited	غير مؤتلف
ἀνατομή	anothomia	dissection	تشريح
ἀντιδιαιρεῖν, ἀντιδιαστέλλειν	contradividere	to be on a par with (in division)	وضع فى القسمة بإزاء
ἀποθεραπευτικός	apotherapeuticus	that provides the completion of the cure	الذى به يتمّ الشفاء
ἁρμονία	armonia	apposition of the surfaces	مطابقة

ἀρτηρία	arteria	artery	شريان ، عرق ضارب
ἄτομοι	atomi	atoms, the indivisible particles	هباء ، الأجزاء التي لا تتجزّأ
αὐχήν	collum	neck	رقبة
βάλανος		suppository	شيافة
βαρυηκοΐα, δυσηκοΐα	difficultas auditus	heaviness of hearing	ثقل السمع
βήξ	tussis	coughing	سعال
βούγλωσσος		bugloss	لسان الثور
γένεσις	generatio	generation, production	حدوث ، تكوّن
γενητός	generabilis	capable of generation	قابل للكون
γενικώτατος	generalissimus	ultimate in the class	لا أعلى منه في الجنس
γένος	genus	class	جنس
τὸ γηροκομικὸν (μέρος)	cirocomica (pars)	geriatrics, treatment of the elderly	تدبير المشائخ
γύψος	gipsum	gypsum	جبسين
δάκτυλος	digitus	finger	اصبع
δέρμα	corium, cutis	skin	جلد
διαγνωστικός	dignoscitivus	recognition	متعرّف
διαίρεσις	divisio	cut	شق
δίαιτα	dieta	diet	تدبير
διαφορά	differentia	class, division, type	صنف
διχίτων	bitunicalis	has two tunics	ذو طبقتين
δύναμις	virtus	force, faculty, power; unguent	قوة ، مرهم
ζωτικὴ δύναμις	virtus vitalis	the animal force	القوّة الحيوانيّة
φυσικὴ δύναμις	virtus naturalis	the natural force	القوّة الطبيعيّة

δυσκρασία	discrasia	defect in the composition	سوء المزاج
δύσπνοια	disnia	defective respiration	سوء التنفّس
ἐγκέφαλος	cerebrum	brain	دماغ
εἶδος	species	form, formation; subdivision	صورة ، نوع
ἕλκος	ulcus	wound, ulcer	جرح ، قرحة
ἐνδεικτικῶς	indicative	indicatively	على طريق الاستدلال
ἔνδειξις	indicatio	deduction, indication	استدلال
ἔντερα	intestina	intestines	أمعاء
καθ' ἕξιν	secundum habitum	firmly rooted	على طريق الثبات والتمكّن
ἐπίδοσις	augmentum	increase	تزيّد ، تزايُد
ἐρυσίπελας	erispila	erysipelas	جمرة
τὸ εὐεκτικόν (μέρος)	euectica (pars)	(the section) which preserves eutrophy; that is concerned with the preservation of eutrophy	حفظ خصب البدن
εὐεξία	euexia	eutrophy	خصب البدن
εὐρυχωρία	spaciositas	interstice	فضاء
ἧπαρ	epar	liver	كبد
τὸ θεραπευτικόν (μέρος)	curativa (pars)	the therapeutic (branch)	(الجزء) الشافي
θεώρημα	theorema	gate of knowledge	باب العلم
ἰός	erugo eris	verdigris	زنجار
ἴς	inulus	fibre	شظية

κακόχυμος	cacochimus	who is suffering from an evil humour	كان فى بدنه خلط ردىء
καρδία	cor	heart	قلب
κατάληψις	cathalipsis, id est comprehensio	comprehension	إدراك
κατασκευή	constructio	state	هيئة
ἐκ καταχρήσεως, καταχρηστικῶς, καταχρώμενος	ex abusione, abusive, abutens	metaphorically	على طريق الاستعارة
κενεαγγίη		emptying of the veins	خلاء العروق
κεφαλαργικός	cephalargicus	who is suffering from a headache	كان فى بدنه صداع
κηλοτόμος	erniarum incisor	who cuts hernias	بطّاط القيل
τὸ κομμωτικόν (μέρος)	commotica (pars)	beauty-treatment	تزيّن للتحسين
τὸ κοσμητικόν (μέρος)	decorativa (pars)	cosmetics, used medicinally	تزيّن طبّىّ
κοτύλη		raṭl	رطل
κράνιον	craneum	skull	قحف الرأس
κρᾶσις	crasis, concretio	composition	مزاج
κρίσις	crisis	crisis	بحران
κύαθος		measure	مكيال
κύστις	vesica	bladder	مثانة
λειεντερία	lienteria	lientery	زلق الأمعاء
λεπτομερής	leptomereus, suptilipartis	with fine parts	لطيف الأجزاء
λήθαργος	litargia	lethargy	السرسام البارد
λιθοτόμος	lapidum incisor	who removes stones	مخرج الحصى
λογικός	logicus	that concerns logic	فى باب من أبواب المنطق
λοῦτρον		bath	حمّام

μέλι	mel	honey	عسل
μελίκρατον		honey water	ماء العسل
ἡ τοῦ ὁμοίου μετάβασις	similis transitio	the switch from one thing to what is like it, differential diagnosis	النقلة (الانتقال) من الشيء إلى نظيره
μῆνιγξ	miringa	mater	أمّ محيط (بالدماغ)
μήτρα	matrix	womb	رحم
μίσυ	vitreolum	vitriol	زاج
μόριον	pars, particula	part, member, limb, tissue	عضو
μῦς	musculus	muscle	عضلة
νεῦρον	nervus	nerve	عصب ، عصبة
νευρώδης	nervosus	belongs to the class of nerves, nerve	من جنس العصب، عصبى
νεφροί	renes	kidneys	كُلَى
ὀδοντικός (ἰατρός)	dentalis (medicus)	dentist	معالج الاسنان
ὀδούς	dens	tooth	سنّ
ὁμοιομερής	omiomerus	homoiomerous	متشابه الأجزاء
ὀξύμελι		oxymel	سكنجبين
ὀξύς	acutus	acute	حادّ
ὀργανικός	organicus	organic	آلىّ
ὄργανον	organum	organ	آلة
ὄρχις		testicle	خصية
ὀστοῦν	os	bone	عظم
οὖς	auris	ear	أذن
οὐσία	existentia, substantia	existence, substance	جوهر ، وجود
ὀφθαλμία	obtalmia	ophthalmia	رمد
ὀφθαλμικός (ἰατρός)	optalmicus (medicus)	oculist	صاحب علاج العين
ὀφθαλμός	oculus	eye	عين
παθητικός	passibilis	liable to pain	قابل للآلام

τὸ παθογνωμονικόν (μέρος)	pathognomonica (pars)	what deals with the forms of disease, deals with the distinction of ailments	صور (تصوير) العلل
τὸ παθολογικόν (μέρος)	passiologica (pars)	pathology	الكلام فى العلل
τὸ παιδοτροφικόν (μέρος)	pedotrofica (pars)	paediatrics	تدبير الصبيان
παράθεσις	iuxtapositio	juxtaposition	تقارب الوضع ، تقارب فى الوضع
παρακεντητής	apunctor	coucher of cataracts	قدّاح الأعين
παρακμή	declinatio	decline	انحطاط
παραφροσύνη	desipientia	mental disorder	اختلاط الذهن
παρέγχυμα	parenchima seu coinfusio	stuffing	حشو
παροξυσμός		crisis, fit	نوبة
παχυμερής	grossiparcius	has thick parts	غليظ الأجزاء
πεπαίνεσθαι		mature	نضج
περιπνευμονία	peripleumonia	pneumonia	ذات الرئة
πιμελή	pinguedo	fat	سمين
πλεύμων	pulmo	lung	رئة
πλευρά	costa	costal	ضلع
πλευρῖτις	pleuritis, pleuresis	pleurisy	ذات الجنب
πληθωρικός	plethoricus	who is suffering from a form of plethory	كان فى بدنه امتلاء
πνεῦμα	spiritus	spirit	روح
ἔμφυτον πνεῦμα	innatus spiritus	the natural spirit	الروح الغريزى
ποτόν		drinking water	ما يشرب
πούς	pes	foot	رجل
πράσιον		leek	ابرسيون
τὸ προγνωστικόν (μέρος)	pronostica, pronosticativa (pars)	prognosis	تقدمة المعرفة ، تقدمة الإنذار ، (الجزء) المنذر

προπαρασκευαστικός	preparativus	preparatory, that first prepares the ground	يتقدّم فيهيّئ، يتقدّم فيعدّ ويهيئ
προσθήκη	adiectio	qualification	استثناء
προταριχεύειν		previously desiccate	سبق فجفّف
τὸ προφυλακτικόν (μέρος)	precustoditiva (pars)	the prophylactic (branch)	التقدّم فى حفظ الصحة
πρωτογενής	primogenitus	the first to be generated	متكوّن بدءا
πτισάνη		barley gruel	كشك الشعير
ῥαφή	sutura	suturing	شأن
ῥῆγμα	scissio	severing	فسخ
ῥητίνη	resina	resin	راتينج
ῥόφημα		broth	حسو
σάρξ	caro	flesh	لحم
τὸ σημειωτικόν (μέρος)	significativa, signativa (pars)	diagnostic (section), diagnosis	استخراج الدلائل ، (الجزء) المستخرج للدلائل
σπάσμα	vulsio	tear	هتك
σπασμός	spasmus	convulsion	تشنّج
σπλήν	splen	spleen	طحال
στέαρ	adeps	tallow	شحم
στερεός	solidus	primary	أصلي
στοιχεῖον	elementum	element	اسطقس، ركن
στοιχειώδης	elementalis	elementary	جار مجرى الاسّطقسات، يجرى مجرى الأركان
κατὰ συμβεβηκός	secundum accidens	in an accidental way	على طريق العرض
συμπάθεια	compassio	communicate the pain	مشاركة فى العلّة
σύνδεσμος	colligatio	ligament	رباط
συνδρομή	concursus	syndrome	اقتران
συστατικός	constitutivus	constitutive	مقوم
σφήνωσις	incuneatio	closure	تغليق

σφυγμός	pulsus	pulse	نبض
κατὰ σχέσιν	secundum habitudinem	as something superimposed	على طريق الإضافة
σῶμα	corpus	body, part, limb	بدن ، جرم ، جسم ، عضو
τελικός	finalis	perfective	متمّم
τένων	tenon	tendon	وتر
τετραφάρμακος	tetrafarmacus	„the Quadruple“	ذو الأربعة الأدوية
τετραχίτων	quadritunicalis	with four tunics	ذو أربع طبقات
τριχίτων	tritunicalis	with three tunics	ذو ثلث طبقات
τύπῳ	figuraliter	sketch	على طريق الرسم
τὸ ὑγιεινόν (μέρος)	sanativa (pars)	preservation of health	حفظ الصحّة ، الحافظ للصحّة
τὸ ὑγρόν	humor	moisture	رطوبة
ὑλικός	materialis	material	موادىّ ، هيولانىّ
ὑμενώδης	membranosus	what belongs to the class of membranes	من جنس الاغشية
ὑμήν	membrana	membrane	غشاء
ὑπερβολή		hyperbole	إغراق
ὑπόχυμα	suffusio	cataract	ماء فى العين
φαρμακεία	farmacia	pharmacy	استعمال الأدوية
τὸ φαρμακευτικόν (μέρος)	farmacalis (pars)	(section that deals with) pharmacy	(جزء) يستعمل الأدوية
φάρμακον	farmacum	drug	دواء
φθαρτός	corruptibilis	capable of corruption	قابل للفساد
φιλοσοφία	phylosophia	philosophy	فلسفة
φιλόσοφος	phylosophus	philosopher	فيلسوف
φλεβοτομεῖν		bleed	فصدَ
φλεβοτομία		bleeding	فصدٌ
φλεγμονή	flegmo	inflammation	ورم ، فلغمونى
φλέψ	vena	vein	عرق غير ضارب ، عرق

φρενῖτις	frenesis	inflammation of the brain	السرسام الحارّ
τὸ φυσιολογικόν (μέρος)	physiologica (pars)	physiology	الكلام فى الأمور الطبيعيّة ، الكلام الطبيعى
τὸ φωνητικόν (μέρος)	vocitativa (pars)	speech training	رياضة الصوت
χαλκός	es	copper	نحاس
χείρ	manus	hand	يد
χειρουργία	cyrurgia	surgery	علاج اليد ، علاج باليد
τὸ χειρουργικόν (μέρος)	cyrurgica (pars)	(section that deals with) surgery	(جزء) يستعمل العلاج باليد
χιτών	tunica	tunic, layer	طبقة ، لباس
χνοώδης	pulverosus	fine dust	فى حدّ الغبار
χόνδρος	cartillago	cartilage	غضروف
χόνδρος		χόνδρος wheat	خندروس
χρεία	utilitas	need, use, useful purpose	حاجة ، منفعة
χρόνιος	cronicus	chronic	مزمن
χυλὸς πτισάνης		barley water, barley gruel	ماء الشعير ، ماء كشك الشعير
χυμός	humor	humour	خلط
ψιμύθιον	cerusa	white lead	اسفيداج
ὠτικός (ἰατρός)	auricularis (medicus)	otologist	معالج الآذان

Bei Fragen zur Produktsicherheit wenden Sie sich bitte an:
If you have any questions regarding product safety,
please contact:

Walter de Gruyter GmbH
Genthiner Straße 13
10785 Berlin
productsafety@degruyterbrill.com